The 10 Best QUESTIONS™

for *Living with Alzheimer's*

The Script You Need to Take Control of Your Health

DEDE BONNER, PH.D.

FOREWORD BY DR. ROGER A. BRUMBACK

A FIRESIDE BOOK
PUBLISHED BY SIMON & SCHUSTER
NEW YORK   LONDON   TORONTO   SYDNEY

DISCLAIMER: This publication contains the opinions and ideas of its author. It is intended to provide helpful and informative material on the subjects addressed in the publication. It is sold with the understanding that the author and publisher are not engaged in rendering medical, health, or any other kind of personal professional services in the book. The reader should consult his or her medical, health, or other competent professional before adopting any of the suggestions in this book or drawing inferences from it.

The author and publisher specifically disclaim all responsibility for any liability, loss or risk, personal or otherwise, which is incurred as a consequence, directly or indirectly, of the use and application of any of the contents of this book.

NOTE: Dr. Dede Bonner and 10 Best Questions, LLC, own the registered trademarks the 10 Best Questions™, the 10 Worst Questions™, and The Magic Question™.

Fireside
A Division of Simon & Schuster, Inc.
1230 Avenue of the Americas
New York, NY 10020

First Fireside trade paperback edition November 2008

FIRESIDE and colophon are registered trademarks of Simon & Schuster, Inc.

For information about special discounts for bulk purchases, please contact Simon & Schuster Special Sales at 1-800-456-6798 or business@simonandschuster.com.

Designed by Mary Austin Speaker

Manufactured in the United States of America

10 9 8 7 6 5 4 3 2 1

Library of Congress Cataloging-in-Publication Data is available.

ISBN-13: 978-1-4165-6051-7
ISBN-10:   1-4165-6051-3

This book is dedicated to my parents, Walter M. and Jane J. Anderson, who knew firsthand about Alzheimer's disease long before it became a household word.

Acknowledgments

I would like to thank the following people who made this book possible: my devoted husband, Randy Bonner; my loving mother, Jane Anderson; my brilliant editor at Simon & Schuster, Michelle Howry; my literary agent, Paul Fedorko of the Trident Media Group; former Simon & Schuster CEO, Jack Romanos; and my attorney, Lisa Davis of Frankfurt Kurnit Klein & Selz, PC, all of whom believed in me and in my vision for the 10 Best Questions series.

I'd also like to thank the experts I interviewed for this book for graciously sharing their time, expertise, and for reviewing my drafts. Please see their biographies in appendix B, "Meet the Experts." My special thanks go to Dr. Roger A. Brumback for his medical expertise and cooperation.

Thanks to my university colleagues, Dr. John P. Fry, Dr. Donald G. Roberts, and Dr. Virginia Bianco-Mathis of Marymount University in Arlington, Virginia; Dr. Cynthia Roman and Dr. Elizabeth B. Davis of The George Washington University in Washington,

D.C.; and Dr. Margaret Novak and Dr. Robert Evans of Curtin University of Technology in Perth, Western Australia.

Lastly, I want to thank all my students in the United States and Australia for their enthusiasm, efforts, and questions. I'd especially like to thank the following students who researched related topics as their class projects and to the experts they interviewed.

From The George Washington University: Diana McChesney and Robin Sharp.

From Curtin University of Technology: Muna Abdullah Al-Raisi, Russell Byrne, Stephen Dunstan, Ashley Hunt, Nanette Jones, Brad Kelly, Mark Latham, Erika Lozano, Sharin Ruba, Balwant Singh, Alan Thornton, Anne Van Den Elzen, John Wareing, and Peter Westlund.

Contents

—

Foreword

————

by Dr. Roger A. Brumback

In his inaugural address of March 4, 1933, President Frank-
lin D. Roosevelt uttered a phrase that has become synonymous
with overcoming adversity: "the only thing we have to fear is
fear itself."

For older individuals (particularly that large group of baby
boomers who are approaching age sixty-five), the "fear" is of inca-
pacitating illness—and the most frightening prospect is disease
that affects the mind. Many boomers have already faced Alzheimer's
disease in their parents or family members; statistics indicate that
Alzheimer's disease is reaching almost epidemic proportions in the
elderly. And now those same boomers are worrying about themselves as well. They wonder, *Is this the normal slower memory I can expect as I get older? Or is it something more sinister?* If you have known
someone with dementia, every memory lapse or momentary mental
slip prompts fear of the early stages of Alzheimer's disease.

Alzheimer's disease (characterized by initial memory loss, followed by loss of other thinking and reasoning abilities) affects one
in ten Americans over the age of sixty-five. What is critically impor-

tant is that a patient—and his or her loved ones and caregivers—
must understand the disease and know how to get the best possible
health care to maximize the quality of life.

Most of the currently available caregiver books written about
Alzheimer's disease (including *Alzheimer's Disease: The Dignity
Within: A Handbook for Caregivers, Family, and Friends*) stress strategies for dealing with the disease by providing examples and anec-
dotes. However, up to now, there has been a major omission in the
available information for patients and families: specifically, how can
a patient and family successfully navigate the health care maze to
assure the best quality of life for the person with Alzheimer's disease? That's where a book like *The 10 Best Questions for Living with
Alzheimer's* comes in.

So how can a book of questions possibly assist in dealing with
Alzheimer's disease? As the famous children's book author Theo-
dor Geisel (better known as Dr. Seuss) said, "Sometimes the questions are complicated and the answers are simple." In order to get
the most help from busy physicians (or other health care providers),
it is necessary for the patient to inquire about the disease and treatment options and to seek clarification about all issues related to the
illness. The only way to do this successfully is for the patient (or
family members) to come to the visit armed with all the questions
that must be answered.

Patients and their families often find it very difficult to formu-
late questions, and even when they do have a list of questions, they
are often too intimidated by the physician to ask the questions
properly. This book simplifies the task, describing how to make the
physician visit less daunting, and how to use questions to optimize
health care decisions. Dr. Bonner has done the complicated work
for you: she's prepared the questions and organized them for easy
use in each step of the path—from the initial diagnosis of Alzheimer's disease to the various treatment and management options.

Knowing the right questions to ask removes some of the anxiety caregivers face in seeking proper health care for their loved one, and allows the patient and family to concentrate on listening to and understanding the answers. Once these questions have been asked and answered, patients and families will be able to use the variety of caregiver books and other resources more successfully to assure a good quality of life for as long a period as possible.

Nothing in life is to be feared, it is only to be understood.
—Nobel Prize winner Marie Curie (1867–1934)

Dr. Roger A. Brumback is Professor of Pathology and Psychiatry and Chairman of the Department of Pathology at the Creighton University School of Medicine in Omaha, Nebraska. Dr. Brumback has trained in pediatrics, neurology (child neurology), anatomic pathology, and neuropathology. He is the founding editor-in-chief of the preeminent Journal of Child Neurology *and has made substantial research contributions in a variety of fields, including genetics, neuropsychiatry, neuromuscular diseases, and cancer. In recent years, his work in Alzheimer's disease has included coauthoring two books for caregivers:* A Caregiver's Guide to Alzheimer's Disease: 300 Tips for Making Life Easier *and* Alzheimer's Disease, The Dignity Within: A Handbook for Caregivers, Family, and Friends *(winner of the* American Journal of Nursing *2006 Book of the Year Award). His Web site is www.rogerbrumback.com.*

Introduction

————

The most important questions are often the ones you didn't know to ask. Even the best doctors in the world can't give you the right answers unless you ask them the right questions first.

But how do you know what the right questions are? "Ask your doctor." You've heard it a million times, but do you *really* know what to ask? What if you don't know very much about Alzheimer's disease yet, feel intimidated by your doctor's expertise, or just feel simply overwhelmed by this diagnosis?

More than ten years ago, when my mother suffered a major heart attack, I felt overwhelmed. As I nervously watched her vital sign monitors bounce around, it occurred to me that I didn't know what to ask the doctors about her condition. In that moment of total helplessness, the only thing I could control was my questions. But I just didn't know what to ask.

I vowed to learn how to ask better questions. When I started taking my mom to her follow-up doctor appointments, I spent time researching her medical options and planning questions for her doctor. I wanted to be a well-informed consumer for her sake so that I could make sure she was getting the very best care possible.

This experience sparked my interest in questioning skills. As I read about questions, I was surprised to learn how little attention most people pay to them. It seems that our society is so focused on solutions and answers that we rarely ever stop to first consider the quality of our questions.

I started teaching questioning skills as part of my graduate-level business classes in Washington, D.C., and Perth, Australia. My students liked it so much that I developed the concept of "The 10 Best Questions" as a way for them to learn questioning skills, team dynamics, and research skills all at once. Since 2003, I've taught hundreds of students who have interviewed thousands of experts. For example, my students have researched what to ask when you buy a house, get engaged, adopt a dog, hire a financial planner, invest in stocks, retire, plan a wedding, start a diet, and have great sex.

To learn more about questions, I conducted a series of interviews with top question askers to understand their secrets. Helen Thomas, the legendary White House reporter, is famous for her press conference questions to every president since John F. Kennedy. She told me, "Before a news conference I would think, What's the best question to ask? I have the courage of ignorance in my questions. I always get nervous, figuring out what to ask a president. But I believe you have to be curious and keep asking why."

Peter Block, an international management consultant and the author of the book *The Answer to How Is Yes,* said, "There's a deeper meaning to asking questions. It's a stance you take in the world, a desire to make contact and get connected."

I talked with many professional interviewers like Susan Sikora, a TV talk show host in San Francisco; New York radio host Debbie Nigro; and Richard Koonce, a journalist and consultant in Brookline, Massachusetts. Each responded with a version of "You are only as good as the questions you ask." For information specific to this book, I also interviewed experts in Alzheimer's, relationships, long-term care, stress, communication skills, financial planning, and caregivers, as well as two former U.S. surgeon generals.

So, who are the best question askers? They are smart, curious, and fearless, yet humble enough to learn from someone else. They value listening and inquiry. Great question askers see every person they meet as a walking encyclopedia of valuable information just waiting to be unlocked by the right questions. And finally, as Albert Einstein once said, "The difference between me and everyone else is my ability to ask the right questions."

The 10 Best Questions in this book won't make you an instant Einstein. And as the Question Doctor, I certainly don't claim any Einstein-like brilliance. I simply believe that a good mind knows the right answers, but a great mind knows the right questions. Now that great mind is yours. This book is "for smarties," not dummies.

Each chapter is a list of the 10 Best Questions derived from as many as 840 questions for that topic and from dozens of books, journals, and Web sites. Each Best Question really had to earn the right to be best by being cited many times. After each question, I've included the "best answers" my experts provided and from my own research so you'll know when you are hearing the full story. The information in this book should not replace medical guidance or professional counseling services.

There is one more question per chapter that I call "The Magic Question." A Magic Question is the one that even smart people rarely think to ask because it's a gut-level question without an obvious answer. Oftentimes, Magic Questions are the ones you think about later and wish you had asked.

In writing this book, I've taken a practical and holistic approach to researching the Best Questions to make you a best-informed patient or caregiver. My focus is to help your key decisions, choices, and relationships by suggesting what you can ask your doctors, medical experts, partner, family, friends, and ultimately yourself after a diagnosis of Alzheimer's disease.

Your lifetime prescription for good health is to stay informed. Former Surgeon General Dr. C. Everett Koop told me in an interview, "There's nothing that will lead to better medical care than a knowledgeable patient." Skip around and read the chapters most relevant to your needs at each stage of the disease.

The 10 Best Questions in this book give you the actual script and best answers in hand for each major conversation and decision you will soon be facing. At the same time, be sure to ask plenty of your own questions, too. As question guru Helen Thomas concludes, "There's no such thing as a bad question, only a lot of bad answers."

The Question Doctor sincerely hopes the Best Questions and answers in this book will give you personal strength and empower you and your loved ones with the knowledge to live as well as possible with Alzheimer's disease.

PART I:

Talking with Your Medical Team

The two most common concerns expressed by newly diagnosed Alzheimer's patients and their families are the fear of the unknown and a fear of not communicating well with their doctors. Your medical team can help you make decisions, but you have to ask the right questions first.

Many people are intimidated by their doctors' knowledge and are reluctant to ask them questions, especially with a diagnosis like Alzheimer's. Use this book to help you. This is no time to be shy, to worry about hurting the doctor's feelings, or to be secretly afraid that he may not "like you" if you ask questions. There's no reason to be aggressive in asking your questions, but be firm in telling your doctor that you expect answers.

To be heard, you may need to repeat your questions or concerns. According to a 1999 study published in *JAMA, The Journal of the American Medical Association,* when patients are trying to talk, doctors typically interrupt after just twenty-three seconds. Persist through interruptions. If your doctor interrupts you before you make your point, try saying "I'd like to finish" or "Can we come back to my concerns later?"

The Best Questions in the first chapter suggest what to ask your doctor when you are first hearing the words "Alzheimer's disease." It assumes that you are talking with your family doctor and are probably too overwhelmed to ask a lot of detailed questions. Chapters 2 and 3 will help you find a top Alzheimer's specialist, while chapter 4 gives you the Best Questions to ask when you're discussing the details of the tests with your new specialist (or family doctor). The last chapter in this section arms you with the Best Questions for getting a second opinion on this diagnosis.

The Question Doctor says, Keep asking questions, both your own and from the following chapters. Even the best doctors can't give you the right answers if you don't ask them the right questions first.

CHAPTER 1: THE 10 BEST QUESTIONS
About a Diagnosis of
Alzheimer's Disease

When I was younger, I could remember anything,
whether it happened or not.

—Mark Twain

Your life is changed forever by a diagnosis of Alzheimer's disease. Some people suspect something is wrong before hearing this news, while others are shocked and overwhelmed to have their worst fears realized for themselves, their aging parent, or their spouse. As Alzheimer's caregiver Jacqueline Marcell, author of *Elder Rage,* says, "Many people are in denial in the beginning. They say, 'We don't want to go to the doctor because it's really not that bad yet. Why do I want to find this out?' "

Seeing your familiar family doctor or a primary care physician may be the easiest way to start getting help. A family doctor who has seen a person regularly for years can recognize subtle changes as the warning signs of dementia, defined as "the progressive decline in cognitive function due to disease and beyond normal aging." Some family doctors prefer to personally conduct the tests and make the initial diagnosis, while others will refer you to a specialist in Alzheimer's disease (also called simply "AD").

Perhaps you are still trying to decide whether or not to see a doctor. If so, ask yourself the following 10 Best Questions to Identify the Warning Signs of Alzheimer's Disease to help your decision. The second list of Best Questions in this chapter provides guidance on what to ask your doctor as you or your loved one is first being told that the diagnosis is Alzheimer's disease.

A well-educated patient and his family have the greatest chance of successfully fighting back the progression of AD for as long as possible. As the high-profile former Surgeon General Dr. C. Everett Koop told this author in an interview, "I always warn people to not think of their questions when they get to the doctor's office but to think of them the day before and write them down."

10 BEST QUESTIONS TO IDENTIFY THE WARNING SIGNS OF ALZHEIMER'S DISEASE

The Alzheimer's Association's list of ten warning signs of Alzheimer's disease has been adapted to the 10 Best Questions format below. See your doctor for a complete evaluation if you or a loved one have several of these signs or are worried about Alzheimer's.

1. **Does the person have a memory loss problem?**
   Even young people have occasional memory lapses. Look for a worsening pattern of forgetting, especially of recently learned information.

2. **Does the person have difficulty performing familiar tasks?**
   Suddenly you or your loved one can't do routine tasks, such as reading the car's fuel gauge, figuring out which coins to give the store clerk, or preparing a favorite recipe.

3. **Does the person have language problems?**
   We all grope for words occasionally, but someone with AD has greater and more frequent difficulty when describing commonplace objects such as a table, toaster, or toothbrush.

4. **Is the person often disoriented about the current time and place?**
   Ask the person for today's date and to tell you the current time on his watch or the hallway clock. Another sign is a person getting lost in her own neighborhood.

5. **Does the person show poor or decreased judgment?**
   Examples include making poor financial decisions, wearing sandals in the snow, or wanting to go shopping at two in the morning.

6. **Does the person have problems with abstract thinking or reasoning?**
   Forgetting how to use numbers, do simple arithmetic, describe objects' appearances, discuss concepts, or solve problems may signal AD.

7. **Is the person frequently misplacing things?**
   Beyond the occasional forgotten car keys, a person with AD may put the phone in the refrigerator, the cereal box in the dishwasher, and the dirty dishes in the car.

8. **Do you notice changes in the person's mood or behavior?**
   People with AD may demonstrate rapid mood swings and different behaviors ranging from sunny calmness to sudden anger to tears for no obvious reason.

9. **Are there changes in his or her personality?**
   Even the sweetest-tempered person with AD can become agitated, paranoid, irritable, fearful, or highly dependent for no obvious reason.

10. **Does the person exhibit a loss of initiative?**
    Alzheimer's disease can cause passivity, depression, and reluctance to do much of anything.

❯❯❯ THE 10 BEST QUESTIONS
About a Diagnosis of Alzheimer's Disease

1. How sure are you that this is really Alzheimer's disease?

This question may be the most important question you ever ask in your life. Most people never think to question a diagnosis of Alzheimer's disease. If your doctor tells you it's Alzheimer's disease, it probably is. But the importance of this Best Question can't be emphasized enough. No matter what, be sure to ask this question. An estimated 10 percent of AD diagnoses are incorrect even with today's improved diagnostic tests.

As Dr. Neill Graff-Radford, a professor of neurology at the Mayo Clinic, explains, "Accuracy is about 90 percent at a good diagnostic center. This means that there's 10 percent that is the wrong type of dementia, not necessarily that 10 percent of people are normal."

Unlike cancer or other diseases that can be diagnosed with great accuracy under a microscope, there is no one single, definitive test for AD. Yet all of your future care and treatment options will hinge on this diagnosis.

Dr. Peter Whitehouse, an experienced Alzheimer's expert and the co-author of the book *The Myth of Alzheimer's,* advises, "You should resist that label and its baggage. Ask, 'What do you mean by Alzheimer's?' "

You have every right to know as much as possible about how this diagnosis was made. This doesn't mean challenging your doctor's personal wisdom or credentials. A good doctor will expect and welcome your questions, especially since total certainty in Alzheimer's diagnoses is impossible until an autopsy after death.

Your brain is far more complex than any other organ. Unlike livers or hearts, which are similar enough among people so that transplants are possible, no two brains are alike. This makes it even more difficult to apply standardized tests to all brains equally. Dr. Roger A. Brumback advises, "A really critical question is, 'How sure are you that this is Alzheimer's or one of the other degenerative dementias and not a treatable condition?' "

A diagnosis of AD should be made only after a whole battery of thoroughly comprehensive medical, neurological, and psychiatric evaluations have ruled out the other causes or types of dementia. Some conditions that masquerade as AD are actually treatable and even curable. These include depression; alcohol; brain tumors; heart, thyroid, or metabolic conditions; head injuries; infections, and vision or hearing difficulties. Drug reactions are a common cause of treatable dementia. Many elderly people are more sensitive to medicines and rely on several different prescriptions, which can cause drug interactions.

In general, the more advanced the dementia is, the easier it is to know with certainty that your loved one has Alzheimer's disease. But if the doctor tells you it's early stage AD or the diagnosis is what's called **mild cognitive impairment (MCI),** insist on more

THE QUESTION DOCTOR SAYS:

Be sure to phrase this question, "How sure . . ." rather than "Are you sure . . ." When you ask a yes/no question like "Are you sure?" you won't get as much information from your doctor as if you had phrased it in a more open-ended way, like "How sure?"

information or get a second opinion. Identifying mild cases of Alzheimer's disease can be very difficult, and doctors don't agree among themselves on what's natural aging memory loss versus a disease.

The bottom line is that you want to make sure up front that you aren't jumping on the Alzheimer's bandwagon when you really don't have a ticket.

2. What type of dementia do you think I have/my loved one has? What is the medical name?

Don't automatically assume a dementia diagnosis is Alzheimer's disease. This is such a well-known household term nowadays that many people—including doctors—are biased toward making this diagnosis.

But there are a surprising number of other dementias, including:

- Mild cognitive impairment (MCI)
- Vascular dementia
- Mixed dementia
- Dementia with Lewy bodies
- Parkinson's disease
- Frontotemporal dementia (Pick's disease, a rare front-temporal neurodegenerative disease)
- Creutzfeldt-Jakob disease

- Normal pressure hydrocephalus
- Huntington's disease
- Wernicke-Korsakoff syndrome

For dementia caused by Alzheimer's disease, there are three types:

1. **Early onset Alzheimer's.** This rare form of AD strikes people younger than sixty-five years old and accounts for less than 10 percent of all AD diagnoses.

2. **Late-onset Alzheimer's.** This is by far the most common form of AD and occurs after age sixty-five.

3. **Familial Alzheimer's disease (FAD).** In this extremely rare type of AD (about 1 percent of cases), the causes are entirely hereditary and onset is usually in the forties.

Ask the doctor to write down the medical name so you can look it up yourself on the Internet or in books for more information.

3. What stage is the disease? What does this mean in my/my loved one's case?

Doctors classify Alzheimer's disease according to the level of cognitive (thinking abilities) and functional (ability to take care of oneself) impairments that a person has. There are two staging systems, one with broad, descriptive categories and the other with seven numerical stages.

The stages of Alzheimer's as classified by descriptive categories are:

Mild. Symptoms include forgetfulness, confusion about time, dates or places, and an increasing inability to perform complex tasks such as planning a calendar, balancing a checkbook, or shopping for groceries.

THE QUESTION DOCTOR SAYS:

Don't forget to ask the last piece of this Best Question, ". . . and what does that mean in my case?" You don't want your doctor discussing general statistics instead of Alzheimer's from the perspective of your or your loved one's unique circumstances, such as age or prior medical conditions.

Mild cognitive impairment (MCI). This new classification is being debated among medical experts as either a form of early AD without functional decline, as a normal aging process, or as a distinct condition. Most, but not all, people with MCI eventually develop Alzheimer's.

Moderate. Now there are noticeable memory problems, difficulties with routine household chores and personal hygiene activities, and personality changes, such as increased irritability.

Severe. The AD person needs continuous care, lacks any awareness, can be incontinent and unsteady on his feet, and shows increased aggression, disorientation, and agitation.

The second classification system for AD uses the following seven numerical stages. See the Alzheimer Association's Web site (www.alz.org) for more details.

Stage 1. Absence of impairment
Stage 2. Minimal impairment
Stage 3. Noticeable cognitive decline
Stage 4. Early stage/mild Alzheimer's
Stage 5. Middle-stage/moderate Alzheimer's
Stage 6. Middle-stage/moderate to late-stage/severe Alzheimer's
Stage 7. Late-stage/severe Alzheimer's

4. What is the prognosis? What can be expected over time? When will I/my loved one die?

This is naturally the first question that jumps to mind for the vast majority of people as they get the initial news about Alzheimer's. However, it is purposely Best Question number 4 so you'll learn more about Alzheimer's before asking it.

Realize that the probable outcome is poor. This disease is characterized by a steady decline until the person is totally disabled. Death normally occurs usually within ten years, and usually from the failure of a body system or an infection.

Every case of AD is different. No doctor can predict the rate of decline because the causes of AD are still unknown and there are many other variables, such as the person's age at onset and her general health. Mayo Clinic's Dr. Graff-Radford says, "The rate of decline varies for each person. Diagnosis to death is very hard to predict."

5. What treatments could I/my loved one benefit from?

This Best Question needs to be asked twice, now when you are first hearing it's Alzheimer's from your family doctor and later during your in-depth meeting with an AD specialist (see Best Question 8 in chapter 4).

At this point, you are probably not ready to hear or understand much about your treatment choices anyway. Give yourself some time to let the diagnosis sink in and the shock wear off. Then you will be ready to learn about your AD drug choices (chapter 6), strategies for staying mentally active (chapter 7), alternative therapies (chapter 8), and clinical trials (chapter 9).

Keep in mind that unfortunately there is no cure for Alzheimer's and that the best you can hope for with any treatment is to slow down the progression of this disease.

6. What will happen if I/we choose to do nothing and not seek treatment? Is that a viable option?

Choosing to do nothing must be a conscious decision reached with your doctor, not a denial of the diagnosis. It's only natural just to want to pretend this diagnosis never happened.

Rather than automatically assuming your best course is to start taking drugs immediately, ask now about likely outcomes if you or your loved one were to just go on with life without treatment of any kind.

All AD treatments only slow the disease, and many are expensive and provide questionable benefits. Doing nothing may be a viable option, depending on the patient's age, prior medical conditions, and other variables such as living and care arrangements. You'll never know unless you ask.

7. How long do I/we have to make decisions about treatments?

Memory deteriorates slowly over years. It's not like everything is normal one day and the next day you have Alzheimer's disease. Even though you may feel panicked at this moment, you may be surprised to hear that you have some time to learn more about Alzheimer's, carefully choose treatments and care options, and to find a top AD specialist or center.

Avoid feeling rushed into hasty decisions from a terrible crush of urgency. As caregiver Elizabeth in Billings, Montana, advises, "Don't overreact. Get support. Try to avoid being sick with worry."

Of course, this timetable depends on your Alzheimer's type, stage, and the guidance you receive from your doctors. Ask your doctors for specific advice in your case.

8. What kind of Alzheimer's specialist do you recommend that we see next?

There is no one kind of doctor who specializes exclusively in treating Alzheimer's. Ask your family doctor or your local chapter of the Alzheimer's Association for names. Chapter 2 gives you the Best Questions to ask once you have referrals and are checking on specific doctors.

The types of Alzheimer's specialists include:

- **Neurologists.** Specialists in nervous system and brain disorders (don't confuse with neurosurgeons, who don't treat AD patients). **Geriatic neurologists** have special training in dealing with elderly patients.
- **Psychiatrists.** Specialists in mental illness.
- **Psychologists.** Specialists in mental illness who aren't medical doctors and can't prescribe medications.
- **Geriatricians.** Specialists in treating illnesses in people over fifty years old.
- **Neuropsychologists.** Specialists in understanding the relationship between the brain and emotional and cognitive functions.

Make your decision based on practical considerations, such as which doctors are covered by your insurance carrier and the doctor's location, as well as your loved one's type of dementia and needs. Keep in mind that not all neurologists, for example, are automatically Alzheimer's specialists. You will probably continue with your family doctor or primary care physician as well after you start seeing an AD specialist.

THE QUESTION DOCTOR SAYS:

Don't ever hesitate to ask other questions that are not in this book. There truly are no dumb questions, especially for a diagnosis with as much uncertainty as the typical early stage AD diagnosis. You have every right to know all the facts about this disease and what it means to you and your family.

9. Where do you recommend that I/my loved one be treated? Why do you recommend this facility? Do they specialize in treating Alzheimer's patients?

Much of the decision about where you get treated will be driven by your choice of specialist and whether you live in a region that is large enough to support specialized AD centers. Be sure to listen to the doctor's reasoning behind her referral.

The worst reason is solely because it's a convenient location. You want convenience, of course, but not if you have to sacrifice high quality standards for AD care and treatment.

10. How can I get more information about Alzheimer's disease? Where can I find emotional and psychological support?

Whether you are the AD patient or the caregiver, you need two kinds of additional information right now, factual and supportive.

Factual information includes details on how the disease progresses and the typical mental and behavioral changes at each stage. There are many books and Web sites available on this topic. See the 10 Best Resources at the end of each chapter and the Resources (page 273) in this book for suggestions.

You also need supportive information to ease your feelings and worries. Again, ask your doctor for his suggestions of the best among the many resources available, including counseling and support groups. The Alzheimer's Association (www.alz.org) is another invaluable place to start.

❯ The Magic Question

What is the most hopeful thing you can tell me about my diagnosis?

Early detection and treatments, especially for MCI and early stage AD, may give you several additional years with a good quality of life. Many people with AD can continue to work and live fairly normally for some time. Research by some of the world's smartest doctors continues as they search for ways to prevent, diagnose, and cure AD.

As Daniel Kuhn of the Alzheimer's Association and author of *Alzheimer's Early Stages* says, "The Alzheimer's label is unfortunately filled with doom and gloom. Many people consider it a death knell, despite the fact there is still much life to be lived. What they need to know is that they can still have a good quality of life. That's the conversation that many physicians don't seem to know how to have."

Ask your doctor for your own good news. AD affects everyone differently, and not everyone progresses at the same rate. Ask about your best possible outcomes, timetable, and prognosis so you can take charge of your life and live it to its fullest now.

CONCLUSION

If your first reaction to a diagnosis of Alzheimer's disease is shock and emotional distress, the next step is to learn as much as you can about your options for treatments and long-term care for you or your loved one.

This diagnosis marks the start of a trip you never asked for or wanted into the world of Alzheimer's disease. Your best strategy for maintaining control of this runaway train is to keep asking your savvy Best Questions all along the way.

THE 10 BEST RESOURCES

Alzheimer's Association. "Basics of Alzheimer's Disease: What It Is and What You Can Do." www.alz.org/national/documents/brochure_basicsof alz_low.pdf.

Alzheimer's Association. "Diagnosing Alzheimer's." www.alz.org/alzhei mers_disease_diagnosis.asp.

Alzheimer's Association. "Early Detection." www.alz.org/alzheimers_ disease_early_detection.asp.

Alzheimer's Association. "Partnering with Your Doctor: A Guide for Persons with Memory Problems and Their Care Partners." www.alz.org/ national/documents/brochure_partneringwithyourdoctor.pdf.

Alzheimer's Association. "Steps to Diagnosis." www.alz.org/alzheimers_ disease_steps_to_diagnosis.asp.

Kuhn, Daniel. "The Need for an Accurate Diagnosis." In *Alzheimer's Early Stages: First Steps for Family, Friends and Caregivers*. Alameda, Calif.: Hunter House Publishers, 2003.

Mayo Clinic. "Alzheimer's Center." www.mayoclinic.com/health/alzhei mers/AZ99999.

MedlinePlus. "Memory." www.nlm.nih.gov/medlineplus/memory.html.

WebMD. "Alzheimer's Disease: Making the Diagnosis." www.webmd .com/alzheimers/guide/making-diagnosis.

Whitehouse, Peter, and Daniel George. *The Myth of Alzheimer's: What You Aren't Being Told About Today's Most Dreaded Diagnosis*. New York: St. Martin's Press, 2008.

CHAPTER 2: THE 10 BEST QUESTIONS

to Get a Reliable Referral for a
Top Alzheimer's Specialist

To know the road ahead, ask those coming back.
—Chinese proverb

If you have been told by your primary care doctor that you or your loved one has Alzheimer's disease (AD), the next step is to find a doctor who specializes in AD treatments and care. Some people prefer to continue seeing their family doctors because they believe AD is a hopeless diagnosis. Others seek a second opinion with a specialist and then go back to their primary care or family doctor.

Most dementia experts believe it's important to see a specialist to confirm the diagnosis. As Dr. Neill Graff-Radford, a professor of neurology at the Mayo Clinic, suggests, "Each patient should have one thorough evaluation at an Alzheimer's center. Experienced doctors are more accurate from a clinical and pathological point of view. A default diagnosis of Alzheimer's disease may be made by doctors less familiar with other diseases."

There is no one specific kind of specialist best qualified to assess and treat AD. Most experts agree, however, that seeing an AD specialist, such as a neurologist, a geriatric psychiatrist, a geriatrician, a psychologist, or a medical practice that specializes in memory disorders, will ensure the best quality of treatments and up-to-date knowledge on the latest AD drugs and research. In any case, you want a top doctor, one that you can trust as a partner during this difficult journey.

You can find an AD specialist by asking your primary care physician, or through family members, friends, an AD support group, or caregivers. If you are like most people, the only questions you probably ask during this brief, initial conversation are to get the new doctor's name, address, and phone number. Perhaps you ask, "Do you like this doctor?" or "Where is he located?" Most likely you trust the person giving you the referral.

In blind faith, you call the prospective doctor's office and schedule the first appointment you can get. As you hang up, you feel a rush of relief because the doctor's receptionist wasn't from Mars and you could get in to see this new doctor quickly.

But you may have just jumped headfirst into potentially dangerous quicksand—and don't even know it. Here's why. It may not have occurred to you that you know virtually nothing about this new doctor. OK, perhaps you did an Internet search or looked him up on various medical Web sites. Yet you have already let slip away your most important ally and information source—the person who already knows him and gave you this referral.

Stop and think about this for just a moment. Here you are on the brink of establishing a very important new relationship with the person who will ultimately hold your health and well-being in his hands. His judgment and experience will be absolutely critical at every step of the way.

Maybe you feel shy about questioning your current doctor closely about his referral, fearful you will somehow insult your doctor's judgment. Maybe you secretly worry your current doctor will think you are dumb or too aggressive if you ask more questions.

Get over it. This is a very important referral and you have every right to know the qualifications of the doctors treating you.

You can't assume that just because you've gotten a referral from your current doctor that this new doctor will automatically be great. There are hundreds of potential reasons behind the referral, ranging from being Friday night poker pals to being long-time partners in the operating room. Caregiver Ellie of Farmington, Michigan, recalls, "I was shocked to learn that my doctor only referred this specialist because they were in the same office complex, but they didn't even know each other." The point is that you just don't know until you ask.

The list of 10 Best Questions below is different than those in the other chapters. It includes questions to ask in two different scenarios. In the first situation, you are asking a medical expert for a referral. Use questions 1 and 2 and The Magic Question when talking with someone with medical expertise.

In the second situation, this time you are getting the referral from current patients or caregivers—your peers. Most doctors' offices will give you the names of several satisfied patients/caregivers whom you can call before you commit to regular visits. When talking with nonmedical people, ask all ten questions below and The Magic Question. As you start, be sure to find out first if this prospective doctor honors your medical insurance.

Don't hesitate to ask. So much is at stake. Having a top doctor with a deep knowledge of AD will make all the difference in your care.

In chapter 3, you'll talk directly to this new doctor. But for now, don't skip this important preliminary step of getting a quality referral first.

>>> THE 10 BEST QUESTIONS
to Get a Reliable Referral for a Top Alzheimer's Specialist

1. Why are you recommending this doctor?

One of the best ways to judge a prospective doctor's quality is through the recommendation from another doctor. Most doctors are sincerely interested in the well-being of their patients and refer them to the doctors they believe offer the best care.

If you are asking a medical professional this question, listen for an answer that includes how impressive this person is in the AD field. Key phrases are "participated in clinical trials" and "presented papers at professional conferences." These are extra-effort activities that earn respect among medical peers. But don't stop there: listen for clues about this prospective doctor's bedside manner as well as his superstar performance at last year's medical conference.

Some doctors fall into referral patterns of always recommending the same doctor down the hallway or a former college roommate. While this isn't necessarily a bad thing, it helps if you know this piece of background information.

If you are talking with caregivers/patients, a good follow-up question is, "How did you originally find this doctor?" If she found this doctor without doing her homework or even worse, from the Yellow Pages, take this person's diminished credibility into account as you assess her answers to your other Best Questions below.

2. How well do you know him or her?

If you are asking a medical professional, you want to hear that they have worked closely together for a number of years. If you are seeking a second opinion, the doctors may not know each other as well, so listen for clues about the prospective doctor's reputation.

Don't assume that someone is a good doctor just because your primary care doctor has referred you to him. You may be shocked to learn they are social friends only and your doctor has little firsthand knowledge about his friend's real doctoring skills.

If you are asking a caregiver/current patient, use this question to make sure it wasn't a short-lived or long-ago relationship that forms the basis of her judgments.

THE QUESTION DOCTOR SAYS:

Be sure to ask open-ended questions, like "How satisfied are you?" rather than "Are you satisfied?" A "how" question will result in much more valuable information than a simple yes/no answer can give you.

3. How satisfied are you with this doctor? In your opinion, what are this doctor's strengths and areas that need improvement?

Depending on this person's degree of openness and willingness to talk, you may get all the details you need by asking simply how satisfied she is.

Ask for descriptions of the doctor's strengths and weakness to help the person giving the referral find the right words to express herself. Be sure to press gently for details on the "areas that need improvement" to understand this doctor's shortcomings. Everyone has shortcomings and this question will help you assess if you can live with this doctor's particular deficiencies or quirks.

4. How well did this doctor communicate with you?

Listen for phrases like:

- I didn't feel rushed when I talked with him.
- He explained everything slowly and used words I could understand.
- He acted like he was really listening to me.
- He made me feel comfortable.
- I could finish my sentences without being interrupted.

5. How well has this doctor kept you informed and encouraged you to ask questions?

This bottom-line Best Question cuts to the core of assessing how patient centered this doctor is. The doctors who are strongly patient centered are more likely to explain treatment options and possible side effects. The best doctors will gladly answer all your questions at any time without exasperation or impatience and will encourage you to learn more about AD.

A doctor who enjoys giving you full and educational explanations is likely to treat you and your loved one with respect. These best doctors encourage their patients to be well informed and to ask questions. In turn, the most knowledgeable patients are usually the most satisfied with their doctors and their care.

6. Did this doctor openly respect your opinions and decisions? Did you ever feel the doctor was talking down to you?

This question helps you to further assess this doctor's attitude toward patients by helping you understand in advance how opinionated he might be when presenting care options. Some people prefer a directive doctor who tells them what to do, while others prefer to do their own research and make independent decisions with the doctor's input.

There's no right or wrong choice along this continuum of personal preferences. Just look for a good match with your own needs and style of communication.

7. How well has this doctor supported you over time?

As the caregiver, you want a doctor who will be your genuine ally during the difficult days ahead. Asking this question now of a person who has already been through the experience is very important. Her answer will go a long way in helping you to set your expectations for quality care and open communications with this particular doctor.

Press gently for more details including how well the doctor handled unexpected complications or advised her about late-stage AD behavioral problems, such as wandering or incontinence. Look for a partner, not just a doctor.

8. Did this doctor include both the caregivers and the patient in the discussions?

This question will help you determine how compassionate and patient centered this doctor is. You want a doctor who values the caregiver's role while respecting the AD patient as a unique individual.

Good indicators are the doctor looking at both the caregivers and patient while explaining something, asking both for questions, and encouraging the caregivers to take notes or make tape recordings of the visit.

9. How accessible was this doctor or office staff after hours or on short notice?

Some doctors are generous with their after-hours time, offering you their cell phone numbers or personal e-mail addresses so you can reach them at any time. Others are not as quick to offer after-hours service. Ask the person giving the referral to share any related stories so you can be realistic about how accessible this doctor will be.

10. How well did this doctor's office staff treat you? Did you ever feel frustrated because of office inefficiency or long wait times to see the doctor?

There's a wide variation in office staff and their responsiveness to patients' needs. You are probably feeling pretty fragile right now, and the last thing you need in your life is a haughty, hostile receptionist or nurse in your doctor's office. You know the one. She acts like it will take an act of divine intervention before she agrees to move two feet to make you a one-page copy for your home files.

You will be depending on this office staff to make sure office appointments are timely, your medical insurance carrier has been properly billed, and to get your loved one's medical records into all the right hands.

❭ The Magic Question

Do you trust this doctor enough to send your own family to her? Why or why not?

This question works well whether you are asking a doctor or a friend for a referral. Trust is an intangible quality and not something that is easily earned.

Just be aware that the response to this "trust test" question is purely subjective. If you don't fully trust the person you are getting the referral from (think Ms. Yellow Pages), be sure to ask the follow-up question, "Why or why not?"

CONCLUSION

By the time you've asked these 10 Best Questions you'll have come a long way, baby, from just getting the prospective doctor's name and number.

You'll know so much more about this doctor's background, strengths, shortcomings, philosophy about patient-centered care, communication skills, and what you can expect in terms of ongoing care and office support.

Think of the person making the referral as a "walking encyclopedia" of valuable information about this prospective doctor. These Best Questions are like the key to unlocking her personal experiences in a way that will be helpful to you without burdening her.

Now you are ready to make your first appointment with a top Alzheimer's specialist. Chapter 3 provides your script for that first visit.

THE 10 BEST RESOURCES

Alzheimer's Association. "Partnering with Your Doctor: A Guide for Persons with Memory Problems and Their Care Partners." www.alz.org/national/documents/brochure_partneringwithyourdoctor.pdf.

American Medical Association. "Making the Most of an Office Visit." In *American Medical Association Guide to Talking to Your Doctor*. New York: John Wiley and Sons, 2001.

Centers for Medicare and Medicaid. "Choosing a Doctor: A Guide for People with Medicare." http://jobfunctions.bnet.com/whitepaper.aspx?docid=121268. (Registration required.)

Consumers' Checkbook. "Medical Advice: Is Your Doctor Measuring Up?" www.checkbook.org. (Subscription required.)

Groopman, Jerome. *How Doctors Think*. Boston: Houghton Mifflin, 2007.

HealthGrades. "Find a Physician." www.healthgrades.com (Charges small fee.)

Manning, Phil R., and Lois DeBakey. *Medicine: Preserving the Passion in the 21st Century*, 2nd ed. Warren, Mich.: Springer, 2003.

National Institute on Aging. "Talking with Your Doctor: A Guide for Older People." www.niapublications.org/pubs/talking/index.asp.

ProHealth's Alzheimer's Support.com. "Starting Your Search." www.alzheimersupport.com/community/referral/#checkup.

Roter, Debra L., and Judith A. Hall. *Doctors Talking with Patients/Patients Talking with Doctors: Improving Communication in Medical Visits*. Westport, Conn.: Auburn House, 1992.

CHAPTER 3: THE 10 BEST QUESTIONS
to Find a Top Alzheimer's Specialist

The *New England Journal of Medicine* reports that nine out
of ten doctors agree that one out of ten doctors is an idiot.

—Jay Leno

ost of us believe that our lives might one day depend on
the right decision by a doctor, a belief we have about
few other professionals. As you face a diagnosis of Alzheimer's disease, that "one day" is no longer abstract. You need Dr.
Right right now.

But before you can proceed, you need to know how to find a really good Alzheimer's specialist. Having a top doctor can make a
world of difference in treatment and care options, behavior management, and your whole quality of life over the next few years.
But how do you find one, especially since there are several different
kinds of specialists? Fear of this potentially scary decision keeps
many families and patients from seeking the specialist care they
need.

When describing their worst experiences with doctors, patients
often cite arrogance, dismissive attitudes, and "callousness," rather
than lack of technical expertise, Ohio State University researchers
found in a 2006 study at the Mayo Clinic. So not only do you need
a technically capable doctor, but also one whom you can feel comfortable with and who will treat you and your need for knowledge
about Alzheimer's disease with respect and dignity.

Dr. Jerome Groopman, in his book *How Doctors Think,* says that
the best doctors have a relish for knowledge, an insatiable curiosity,
pride in their performance, and a "clear, clean joy in sharing with
you [their] knowledge." He cites among the worst attributes a

THE QUESTION DOCTOR SAYS:

Be sure to tell your doctor at the beginning of your appointment that you have a list of questions and ask when she prefers to answer them. This way you'll know her preference for timing and will have politely informed her that you want enough time to get your questions answered.

doctor's unwillingness to listen, cynicism, and the tendency to treat all patients the same with "cookie cutter" or one-size-fits-all treatments.

Even if you prefer to stay with a family doctor for ongoing Alzheimer's care, you owe it to yourself to seek at least a second opinion (which is often covered by insurance carriers) from an Alzheimer's specialist so you can avoid future regrets and doubts.

The 10 Best Questions in this chapter will help you with this important task. Again, the best doctors will welcome your questions and your desire to choose doctors carefully. If a doctor reacts negatively to your questions or refuses to answer, see this as a red flag that the doctor either has something to hide or that she may be impatient with you during future office visits.

>>>THE 10 BEST QUESTIONS
to Find a Top Alzheimer's Specialist

1. Are you board certified? What are your other medical credentials?

Board certification matters.

Board certification assures you that the doctor has passed the requirements of certification for her specialty. In the United States, medical specialty certification is voluntary. Doctors receive their medical licenses after completing medical school. But to be a spe-

THE QUESTION DOCTOR SAYS:

If you feel shy or intimidated about asking a potential doctor about credentials, ask the office staff, go to the doctor's Web site or bio, or simply do your own search using the resources in this chapter. If you are satisfied about a doctor's credentials, skip asking this question in person. But don't skip this Best Question altogether just because it seems hard to ask. You don't want someone who has served jail time for malpractice prescribing medications for your loved one!

cialist like a neurologist, the doctor does additional training called a residency. After completing the residency training, a doctor can apply for certification by a specialty board.

Successful completion of the examinations to complete board certification demonstrates a doctor's exceptional expertise and her dedication to a rigorous, voluntary commitment to lifelong learning. This is especially important with Alzheimer's disease because doctors need to stay current with the fast-moving research advances in this field. To maintain board certification, doctors must complete yearly training and take periodic exams to demonstrate their ongoing competency. Use the search services of the American Board of Medical Specialties (www.abms.org) to check for a specific doctor's certification.

A valid state license is also very important. Go to the American Medical Association's Web site (www.ama-assn.org) and click on your state for specific information about a doctor you are considering. Links to state boards are available at www.ama-assn.org/ama/pub/category/2645.html.

Checking on past disciplinary actions and malpractice suits is tougher because most medical professionals don't readily disclose unclean histories. See ChoiceTrust (www.choicetrust.com) or HealthGrades (www.healthgrades.com), two comprehensive Web sites that charge a small fee for their searchable services. Other sources for checking on prior complaints or disciplinary actions are free at Administrators in Medicine (http://docboard.org) and Health Care Choices (www.healthcarechoices.org).

2. What is your experience with Alzheimer's patients? How many Alzheimer's patients did you see during the past twelve months?

Experience matters, too. The number of years of total medical practice is significant, along with the years of specialized practice a doctor has in treating Alzheimer's disease.

It's very important to determine a doctor's prior experience with Alzheimer's. One way to determine a doctor's specialized expertise is to ask this follow-up question: "What percentage of your practice is devoted to treating Alzheimer's patients?" The higher the better. You also want to ask, "How many total times have you treated Alzheimer's disease?" (Alzheimer's disease was rarely diagnosed correctly before the mid-1980s.)

If you live in a rural community or have limited access to specialized care centers, doctors will naturally have lower yearly numbers. In this case, ask this Best Question as a percentage of this doctor's total practice, like, "What percentage of your patients are Alzheimer's cases?" in addition to getting a total number.

A good bedside manner can be very comforting. But don't choose a doctor based on his personality alone. A doctor's personality should be your secondary—not the primary—consideration in making your choice.

3. May I speak to at least one of your patients to see how he or she made out in these same circumstances?

This Best Question was suggested by former Surgeon General Dr. C. Everett Koop. He believes it's very important to follow through on patient referrals.

Asking for a referral is more common than you might think. Chapter 2 gives you specific Best Questions for getting highly reliable referrals.

4. Which hospitals are you affiliated with?

Although early stage Alzheimer's patients rarely need hospitalization (except for treating other medical conditions), this answer could be very important later.

You have two choices. You can choose your doctor first and then go with the hospital where she has admitting privileges. Or you can choose the hospital or Alzheimer's facility first and then find a top doctor there.

In the second scenario you are focused on the facility's expertise or reputation first over an individual doctor's skills. Either way, ask this follow-up question; "What is the accreditation status of this medical facility?" See The Joint Commission's Web site (www.jointcommission.org) for more on accreditation.

5. Are you affiliated with any medical schools?

A teaching affiliation with a prestigious medical school is the gold standard when looking for a top specialist. It's a fairly reliable indicator that a doctor is considered by her peers to be a leader in the Alzheimer's field.

Academic doctors who also practice medicine are likely to be the most well informed about the latest in Alzheimer's research, diagnostic tools, and treatments and they will keep current through frequent contacts with their medical colleagues.

6. Are you involved with any ongoing research projects or clinical trials on Alzheimer's disease?

Experts suggest that you look for doctors who have written about AD and whose work is often cited in medical journals.

If a doctor you are considering has been published, ask for copies of those articles. Even if the articles are full of jargon or boring, you can learn a lot about this doctor's interests and approach to treating Alzheimer's. Go to PubMed Central (www.pubmed central.nih.gov) for a free archive of medical journal abstracts.

7. Are you part of a team that holds regular meetings to discuss patients' cases and treatments?

Doctors often emphasize how important a multidisciplinary team behind the scenes is for ensuring quality patient care, accurate diagnoses, and effective treatment plans. More heads are better than one in making accurate and well-informed diagnoses and providing better patient care.

Doctors practicing in teaching hospitals or large Alzheimer's centers are more likely to be part of a team. Not having this team approach isn't necessarily a deal breaker, but it's good if you can get it.

8. How will you keep my family involved in care decisions? Do you offer support services and more information about Alzheimer's disease?

The doctor's answer to this question will give you a great insight into how patient centered and family centered she really is. You want a doctor who considers you and your family as unique individuals.

If you have choices, go to a doctor who offers support services, such as specially trained geriatric nurses, physical therapists, nutritionists, and family counselors. At later stages you'll have these other needs for which a family-centered specialist can be a godsend.

The best doctors are also good teachers at heart. As retired acting Surgeon General Rear Admiral Dr. Kenneth P. Moritsugu comments, "When the doctor seeks to educate the patient, they are not merely engaging in a two-way conversation. Rather, the doctor is taking it beyond the conversation in order to teach the patient about medical options and how to take control of his or her own health and well-being."

9. Please describe your preferences for communicating with your patients.

Communication obstacles rank high on patients' list of complaints. Most people highly value how well a doctor communicates with both the patient and his family, especially since Alzheimer's primary caregivers are so directly and personally involved with the patient's well-being.

10. Who covers for you when you aren't available or are on vacation?

This is another question that most patients don't think to ask until they can't reach their doctor when they need to.

Be sure that your doctor tells you how she will communicate with you if unanticipated problems come up or when she's unavailable or on vacation. A follow-up question is to ask how (calls or e-mails) and when (best times of day) she can be reached.

❯ The Magic Question

What is the last thing you learned about Alzheimer's disease?

The best answer to this question is not so much what the doctor says, but how easily the response rolls off her tongue.

If this doctor is truly an excellent doctor and sees plenty of AD patients, she'll be able to easily say something like, "Well, I read an article last week" or "I went to a conference last month." But if she is groping for an answer, look elsewhere for your AD specialist. You don't want her to be the last one to know about new Alzheimer's research discoveries and improved drugs.

CONCLUSION

If a prospective doctor obviously enjoys—passionately enjoys—the practice of medicine, shows evidence of following new developments, obviously thinks hard about you and your problems, asks questions of you, shows a real interest in your answers, and meets the requirements for board certification and experience, you probably have a good doctor. From the group of good doctors you find, choose one you can trust and feel comfortable with.

Dr. Roger A. Brumback concludes with this observation: "Alzheimer's disease really requires a specialist's evaluation. No one should walk away from a doctor's office with the diagnosis 'Well it's *probably* Alzheimer's disease' without having a full examination by a highly competent doctor."

THE 10 BEST RESOURCES

Consumers' Checkbook. "Guide to Top Doctors." www.checkbook.org. (Subscription required.)

Consumers Union of U.S. "Doctor, Can We Talk? How to Develop a Good Relationship with a New Physician." Special Report for *Consumer Reports On Health*. July 2001.

Groopman, Jerome. "Epilogue: A Patient's Questions." In *How Doctors Think*. Boston: Houghton Mifflin, 2007.

HealthGrades. "Find a Physician." www.healthgrades.com. (Charges small fee.)

Leeds, Dorothy. *Smart Questions to Ask Your Doctor*. New York: Harper Paperbacks, 1992.

Manning, Phil R., and Lois DeBakey. "Reading: Keeping Current." In *Medicine: Preserving the Passion in the 21st Century*, 2nd ed. New York: Springer, 2003.

Morris, Virginia, and Robert M. Butler. "Doctor Do's and Don'ts." In *How to Care for Aging Parents*. New York: Workman Publishing, 2004.

National Institute on Aging. "Talking with Your Doctor: A Guide for Older People." www.niapublications.org/pubs/talking/index.asp.

Radin, Lisa. "Finding the 'A' Team." In *What If It's Not Alzheimer's: A Caregiver's Guide to Dementia.* Amherst, N.Y.: Prometheus Books, 2003.

U.S. News and World Report. "Best Hospitals 2007 Specialty Search: Neurology and Neurosurgery. http://health.usnews.com/usnews/health/best-hospitals/search.php?spec=ihqneur. (Updated annually.)

CHAPTER 4: THE 10 BEST QUESTIONS

About the Test Results for
Alzheimer's Disease

It's not over until it's over.

—Yogi Berra

Y<span></span>ou've been told that you or your loved one probably has Alzheimer's disease. Perhaps your family is feeling sad, angry, and afraid. If so, one way to move beyond your emotional reactions is to sharpen your mind about what this diagnosis really means and try to learn more about Alzheimer's disease.

This book assumes that you've talked with your family doctor, who suspects it's Alzheimer's, asked around for a reliable referral, chosen an Alzheimer's specialist, and now you are getting ready to meet with your new specialist to discuss the results of the various tests that he requested to confirm a diagnosis of Alzheimer's disease. Even if this is not your actual experience or chronology, you'll still want to know more about what the tests have revealed by asking your AD specialist or family doctor specific questions.

There is no one single, simple test for AD. Your evaluation should have included a full medical history, a complete physical examination, multiple blood chemistry and laboratory tests, neuropsychological testing to assess memory and other cognitive functions, and a brain-imaging scan. The overall goal of a diagnostic workup is to explore every possible cause of a person's symptoms and to determine if the memory loss is caused by a condition that is reversible or treatable. Since doctors can't directly observe the workings of your brain, many of these tests are done to rule out other medical conditions in a process of elimination before calling it Alzheimer's. That's why having a whole series of different tests is so important.

Understanding these tests is critical. They hold the key to the diagnosis, prognosis, and treatment plan. During this important office visit you and your doctor may make key decisions on future treatment and care choices based on these test results.

But most people are clueless on what to expect or what to ask. Many feel overwhelmed. Knowing in advance the Best Questions for this meeting with your doctor will give you a sense of control and help you move from being a passive victim of this dreaded disease to being a more active player with your medical team. Note that the advertised home screening tests now available are not recommended by the Alzheimer's Association as a reliable substitute for a full professional medical review.

Experienced caregivers and patients advise you to bring along another family member as a pair of listening ears, along with a notepad and even a tape recorder to this appointment. If your loved one with Alzheimer's is likely to be restless or resistant during the appointment, consider bringing a third person who can manage his behavior so you can give the doctor your full attention.

THE QUESTION DOCTOR SAYS:

Find out how your doctor prefers to deal with questions, either before, during, or after his explanation of the test results. This small courtesy will build a good relationship with your doctor, while letting him know your intention to take an active role in this discussion and decisions.

Don't be afraid to learn more about Alzheimer's disease. It's what you don't know that can hurt you. No one expects you to be a medical genius. All you need are the right questions. Let your doctors come up with the right answers. Be sure to ask your own additional questions, too.

>>>THE 10 BEST QUESTIONS
About the Test Results for Alzheimer's Disease

1. Which tests were done? Please summarize the tests that have been performed to date. Are additional tests needed?

It is likely that your loved one had a comprehensive examination that involved several types of evaluations and may have taken more than one day in several locations. There are four types of tests commonly performed: (1) medical history and physical examination, (2) laboratory blood and urine tests, (3) neuropsychological (memory and thinking) tests, and (4) brain imaging tests.

Ask for a copy of any written reports or images, especially if you will be seeking a second opinion or going back to your family doctor for long-term medical care. The next four Best Questions below cover each of these four types of tests. Be sure also to ask if additional tests will be needed now or in the future. If so, ask why.

2. What did the medical history and physical exam reveal?

The medical history is assembled through interviews or a questionnaire to identify the patient's current and past medical problems, difficulties in daily activities, prescription drug use, and any family history of dementia or other mental conditions.

The doctor may also interview close family members for supplemental information, such as the patient's emotional and mental state, past head injuries, and associated symptoms like depression, insomnia, incontinence, delusions, hallucinations, verbal, emotional or physical outbursts, sexual disorders, and weight loss.

The physical examination should be thoroughly comprehensive and include evaluations of hearing and sight, reflexes, sensation, strength, balance, and coordination, readings of the heart, lungs, blood pressure, pulse, and strength of grip, an EEG (electroencephalogram or brain wave test), and detailed questions about the patient's diet, exercise, and use of alcohol.

3. What did the laboratory tests reveal?

Laboratory tests and the collections of blood and urine samples are analyzed to eliminate any other possible causes of memory loss and confusion, such as malnutrition, a urinary tract infection, or drug side effects. These blood chemistry tests include a complete blood count (CBC), tests of thyroid, kidney, and liver and immune system function, and tests for vitamin deficiencies, anemia, glucose levels, and other indictors of illness that can be determined with blood tests. Sometimes spinal fluid is collected for testing to rule out specific disorders of the nervous system.

Ask the doctor to review with you the results of each laboratory test. As a follow-up question, ask what your loved one's specific numerical results are and what the normal range is for that test. If the result is normal, ask if there are any "high normals" or borderline numbers.

4. What did the mental status tests reveal?

Formal neuropsychological testing involves a battery of standardized tests of memory and thinking to assess the person's awareness of having symptoms, his sense of orientation in time, place, and balance, and his ability to recall, complete, or generate short lists of words.

One of the most common tests is called the Mini–Mental State Exam (MMSE), in which the person is asked questions like the current date, the names of common objects, and to count backward. Results are compared to normal people of similar age and education. The MMSE is not a formal neuropsychological test and should not be the only neuropsychological functioning test used to make a diagnosis. The maximum MMSE score is 30, with a score of 20–24 indicating mild dementia, 13–20 moderate dementia, and under 12 indicating severe dementia. Ask for your loved one's score.

The MMSE test is simple and used by many general practitioners. But it isn't considered as sophisticated as other mental function tests like the Alzheimer's Disease Assessment Scale (ADAS-cog). Additional tests used to diagnose early-stage dementia are the Blessed Information-Memory-Concentration Test, the Blessed Orientation-Memory-Concentration Test, and the Short Test of Mental Status.

A well-qualified neurologist will be familiar with a wide variety of other tests for assessing problem solving, abstract thinking, attention, and vision-motor coordination and will choose the most appropriate assessments for each individual. A screening evaluation for depression/anxiety conducted by a geriatric psychiatrist is also important because depression can cause reversible memory loss.

5. What were the results of the brain imaging tests?

Brain-imaging scans are now commonly used to eliminate the possibility of brain tumors, strokes, or blood clots in the brain as the reason for symptoms. These detailed pictures of the brain include CT scans (computerized tomography), MRIs (magnetic resonance imaging), PET scans (positron emission tomography), and SPECT scans (single-photon emission computerized tomography).

Brain images will reveal any changes in the brain structure or size that are characteristic of Alzheimer's disease as well as help your doctor exclude other causes of dementia, such as a tumor or stroke. Some people with early stage AD have normal brain images.

6. How sure are you that this is Alzheimer's disease? What specifically (test results, etc.) makes you so sure?

You are repeating this most critical question again, this time with an AD specialist rather than your family doctor or primary care physician. Make sure this doctor gives you a full explanation, including specific sections of the tests results that indicate Alzheimer's and not another disease. The importance of asking this question again can't be overemphasized.

According to the Alzheimer's Association, experts estimate that a skillful doctor can diagnose AD correctly in 85 to 90 percent of his cases. However, that's still 10 to 15 percent of people who are told they have Alzheimer's but have actually been misdiagnosed—and may never know it. Alzheimer's is just one kind of the many dementias. Other conditions can also cause similar symptoms.

Keep in mind that every diagnosis of Alzheimer's is probable and not definite. If you or your doctor has even a small margin of doubt, strongly consider getting a second (or third) opinion or ask for additional tests. A good doctor will welcome your insistence for certainty and good detective work and not be threatened or offended by this question.

Dr. Peter Whitehouse, the co-author of *The Myth of Alzheimer's*, says, "I find very few experts in this field who truly believe this is a singular condition contrasted to multiple processes or causes. And yet, we always use the singular. There are many, many people who recognize that the overlaps with normal aging are great."

7. What type of AD does my loved one have? What is the stage (extent) of his Alzheimer's disease?

You may have already been told by your family doctor or during an earlier doctor's visit your loved one's type and stage of Alzheimer's disease. (See chapter 1, Best Questions 2 and 3.) The three types of

AD are early onset, late-onset, and familial Alzheimer's disease. The stages are described as early, moderate, or severe, with mild cognitive impairment (MCI) sometimes classified separately or along with early stage Alzheimer's.

The other, more detailed, seven-stage system for AD is:

Stage 1. Absence of impairment
Stage 2. Minimal impairment
Stage 3. Noticeable cognitive decline
Stage 4. Early stage/mild Alzheimer's
Stage 5. Middle-stage/moderate Alzheimer's
Stage 6. Middle-stage/moderate to late-stage/severe Alzheimer's
Stage 7. Late-stage/severe Alzheimer's

8. Please explain my/my loved one's treatment options.

This discussion is aimed at starting a dialogue with your doctor to map out a treatment plan. You'll have more detailed discussions later about drugs and other treatment choices, but for now you want general guidelines on what you can reasonably expect for both the short-term and long-term progression of your loved one's disease.

A strong follow-up question is to ask now is if there are any feasible treatments that don't involve medications, also known as alternative treatments, complementary/alternative medicine, or integrative medicine. Part II of this book provides specific Best Questions for making well-informed treatment choices.

9. Am I/my loved one a good candidate for participating in a clinical trial?

If you are potentially interested in participating in a clinical trial, ask your doctor if he thinks you or your loved one would be a good candidate, and if so, when you need to make a decision. Sometimes patients and families need to make decisions fairly early in the treatment process. See chapter 9 for the Best Questions on this topic.

10. Can I/my loved one continue to drive safely? To go to work? To live alone or independently? To carry on my/his normal daily activities? If so, for how long?

Understanding realistically what changes to anticipate in daily activities will help you tremendously now and later as you are planning for a future with this progressive disability. Remember that for many with early stage AD or MCI, their mental decline is a slow process and they can continue to function fairly normally, at least for a while.

Try to learn everything you can from your doctor about the timeline for you or your loved one's growing dependence on a caregiver. At the same time, realize that even the best doctor can't predict with total certainty the rate of decline in your or your loved one's case.

Ask for additional resources to read and people to talk with. Contact the Alzheimer's Association for additional guidance on living with AD. You might also want to inquire about the services of an occupational, rehabilitation, or physical therapist to evaluate your or your loved one's **Activities of Daily Living (ADLs)** to determine how well he can still do the simple tasks (fix a meal, dress himself, etc.) associated with independent living.

❯ The Magic Question

Under what circumstances should I/we contact your office?

This is a question few people think to ask in advance.

Rather than you trying to figure out what changes in your loved one's mental functioning or behavior are important enough that you call for an appointment or take him to the hospital's emergency room, ask your doctor now. Your doctor will help you sort out the differences between a serious situation that requires medical attention and your possible overreaction to events. Typical reasons to contact the doctor immediately include:

- Sudden increase in confusion
- Blackouts, fainting, falls, or fever
- Sudden inability to talk or move
- Onset of accidents or wetting the bed
- Major change in memory or mood swings

This question is another way of asking your doctor to help you understand his definition of "normal" for your loved one's type and stage of AD in between doctor visits.

CONCLUSION

Your doctor should seek irrefutable evidence of your loved one's pattern of declining memory in order to make a diagnosis. This includes a highly detailed and focused personal, medical, mental, and physical history assessment. Brief mental status tests are useful but should not be used as the only diagnostic tool. Author and pathologist Dr. Roger A. Brumback, says, "There are a lot of situations where the diagnosis is never challenged."

The bottom line goal is for both you and your doctor to be very, very sure that this is Alzheimer's disease. Learn everything you can about AD along the way and let your doctors educate you by giving you their best answers to your Best Questions. Dr. Peter Whitehouse says in his book *The Myth of Alzheimer's,* "We don't even know how to diagnose Alzheimer's disease, let alone tabulate the numbers of disease victims. Because there is no single biological profile for AD, every clinical diagnosis is considered 'probable.'"

THE 10 BEST RESOURCES

Alzheimer's Association, "Conducting an Assessment." www.alz.org/pro fessionals_and_researchers_conducting_an_assessment.asp.

Alzheimer's Association, "Steps to Diagnosis: Reviewing Medical History." www.alz.org/alzheimers_disease_steps_to_diagnosis.asp.

Doerflinger, Deirdre M. Carolan. "Mental Status Assessment of Older Adults: The Mini-Cog," *Try This,* November 2007. Hartford Institute for Geriatric Nursing. www.hartfordign.org/publications/trythis/issue03.pdf..

Fisher Center for Alzheimer's Research Foundation. "Alzheimer's Diagnosis Importance." www.alzinfo.org/alzheimers-diagnosis.asp.

Manning, Phil R., and Lois DeBakey. "Evidence-based Medicine." In *Medicine: Preserving the Passion in the 21st Century,* 2nd ed. New York: Springer, 2003.

Mayo Clinic. "MRI: Viewing Your Brain and Other Soft Tissues." www .mayoclinic.com/health/mri/SM00035.

National Institute on Aging. "Talking to Patients About Cognitive Problems." www.nia.nih.gov/HealthInformation/Publications/Working withYourOlderPatient/chapter10.htm.

Revolution Health. "Diagnosing Alzheimer's: An Interview with a Mayo Clinic Specialist." www.revolutionhealth.com/conditions/brain-nerves/alz heimers/diagnosis/diagnose-interview.

Timmermans, Stefan, and Marc Berg. *The Gold Standard: The Challenge of Evidence-Based Medicine.* Philadelphia: Temple University Press, 2003.

Whitehouse, Peter, and Daniel George. "Preparing for a Doctor's Visit." In *The Myth of Alzheimer's*: What You Aren't Being Told About Today's Most Dreaded Diagnosis. New York: St. Martin's Press, 2008.

CHAPTER 5: THE 10 BEST QUESTIONS

to Ask When Getting a Second Opinion

Every road has two directions.

—Russian proverb

A 2001 research report by the Alzheimer's Association called the *Alzheimer's Disease Study: Communication Gaps Between Primary Care Physicians and Caregivers* concluded that the majority of caregivers who suspected a family member or close friend had Alzheimer's went to their primary care physician (PCP) first. However, the study found surprisingly wide discrepancies between the caregivers' opinions about how well their doctors communicated and how well the PCPs thought they were communicating. For example, compare the 38 percent of caregivers who believe their PCPs actually provided the information they needed with the 83 percent of PCPs who believed they had adequately informed their patients about AD.

If you or your loved one is facing a diagnosis of Alzheimer's disease, there are three key reasons to consider getting a second opinion. First, AD is a complex, life-threatening disease. This diagnosis will change both the patient's and her family's lives forever.

Second, every diagnosis of Alzheimer's is considered "probable" because there is no definitive test for it. In addition, every person with AD has a different progression, time frame, and behavior pattern.

And third, many insurance carriers will pay for a second and sometimes even a third opinion for Alzheimer's disease. Check with your health care provider for their specific policies beforehand.

Dr. Vicki Rackner, a patient advocate, board-certified surgeon, and author, is a strong believer in the value of second opinions. She says simply, "You need a second opinion for everything."

Pathologist Dr. Roger A. Brumback agrees. He says, "Second opinions of a diagnosis of Alzheimer's disease are becoming more common but it needs to be a universal practice."

Caregiver advocate and author Jacqueline Marcell also believes in the value of second opinions. She says, "Getting a second opinion and making sure you are talking with a dementia specialist, like a neurologist specializing in dementia, is really important. There are so many types of dementias. You need to know what to expect going forward and get the best care possible."

You especially need a good-quality second opinion if you've only seen your family doctor or a primary care physician so far. The other circumstances where a second opinion is most warranted are if the diagnosis is either mild cognitive impairment (MCI) or early stage AD. Both of these conditions are more difficult to diagnosis with high certainty than moderate or late-stage AD.

You may be undecided about whether or not you really need a second opinion, especially if you must pay for it yourself. If that's your situation, ask *yourself* the first five Best Questions below to help you decide what to do.

If you've already decided that you do want a second opinion, first find another doctor using the Best Questions in chapters 2 and 3. Once you have this new doctor, use Best Questions 6 through 10 in this chapter to guide your discussion with the second-opinion doctor.

>>> THE 10 BEST QUESTIONS
to Ask When Getting a Second Opinion

Best Questions to Ask Yourself *Before Getting
a Second Opinion*

1. How do I rate my current doctor's knowledge about Alzheimer's disease and his ability to support me and my family during our loved one's decline?

The Alzheimer Association study cited at the beginning of the chapter found that caregivers underestimate what they should know about AD and its treatment. At initial diagnosis, you probably still don't know that there are many more complexities to treating Alzheimer's than it would first appear. Primary care physicians may know about AD, but they were not effectively communicating that knowledge, according to this study.

No doubt AD specialists, including neurologists, geriatric psychiatrists, geriatricians, and psychologists, will be more knowledgeable than a primary care physician. You want a doctor you can count on through your loved one's progressive AD stages.

2. How confident am I in my current doctor's interest in treating me and my loved one as unique persons?

Think back to your doctor's treatment plan for your loved one. How comprehensive was it? Did she seem sincerely interested in both of you as individuals? Did she discuss a range of treatments to try? Do you feel you can trust her?

By all means, avoid doctors who only prescribe the same drugs over and over again. Legendary psychologist Abraham Maslow once noted that when all you have is a hammer, everything looks like a nail. The same applies here. When a doctor only knows a small handful of treatment options, every patient looks the same—like a nail with Alzheimer's disease.

3. How much do I/we understand about what I've/we've been told to date about the Alzheimer's diagnosis and treatment options?

Reflect on your prior discussions with your doctor. Look over your notes and listen to tape recordings of your prior medical appointments.

Confer with other family members who accompanied you to medical appointments and compare your impressions. Scan this book to learn more about the various types of treatments. All of this will help the factual information to sink in as you step back to assess your situation for a moment.

Now with this cleared head, think through logically how much you truly understand. This is not a reflection of your intelligence, but rather a sign of how well the AD diagnosis and treatment plan has been explained to you. You want a doctor who is willing and capable of putting medical jargon into easy-to-understand terms for you and your family.

The word "doctor" is from the Latin *docere*, meaning "to teach." The medical profession has evolved over time and now we think of doctoring and teaching as two separate functions. But look for a good doctor who is also willing to be your teacher.

4. How complicated is my/my loved one's diagnosis and treatment plan?

Don't assume that just because there's no cure for Alzheimer's disease, it's time to throw in the towel. Many people with early stage AD continue to live full lives, especially if they embrace healthy living habits with better diet, exercise, and mental activities.

Ideally, you want a doctor who stays current on the latest breakthroughs in Alzheimer's research and care. Even if your loved one has what seems to be straightforward AD, there's still much to learn, as well as many treatment decisions and care choices to discuss with your doctor in the future.

5. What does my inner voice tell me is right for me?

There's a lot to be said for the value of going with your gut-level reaction. This question suggests that after you've asked all the highly logical, rational, analytical questions, you should also listen to your inner voice.

Malcolm Gladwell, the author of *Blink,* would agree. He says, "We really only trust conscious decision making. But there are moments, particularly in times of stress, when haste does not make waste, when our snap judgments and first impressions can offer a much better means of making sense of the world."

THE QUESTION DOCTOR SAYS:

Use these following five Best Questions to ask a second doctor if you are seeking an AD specialist, a second opinion on the diagnosis or treatment plan, or just to find a doctor you'll like better. Before you begin your doctor search, get a clear idea of what kind of doctor you want and why.

Best Questions to Ask the Doctor *When Getting a Second Opinion*

6. How do you interpret my/my loved one's test results?

Ask the second doctor to review the test results to give you his interpretation of the diagnosis.

Medical experts and families disagree about whether your second opinion should be "blind." A blind second opinion means that the first doctor's opinion and sometimes the original test results aren't shared with the second doctor.

The advantage is that the blind second opinion will be more objective and not influenced by the first one. The drawbacks include putting your second opinion doctor at a disadvantage by not letting him know the basis for the original diagnosis. Another option is to provide test results and other information without including the first doctor's diagnosis and recommendations on treatment.

7. What are the chances that the test results could indicate a different diagnosis?

Statistically, you have at least a one in ten chance that the second doctor will determine a different diagnosis.

Dementia is expressed in highly individual ways among people suffering from memory loss. The milder the dementia (such as MCI or early stage AD), the greater the probability that your original diagnosis was incorrect.

8. In your opinion, has my/my loved one's Alzheimer's disease been properly diagnosed? Please explain the rationale for your answer.

This is a straightforward question that goes to the heart of why you want a second opinion. Make sure the second doctor takes the time to fully explain the reasoning behind her assessment of your or your loved one's symptoms.

Don't hesitate to ask any other questions so you can understand what you're being told in response to this question.

9. Are there any alternative forms of treatment available that my previous doctor may have overlooked? What treatments do you recommend for me/my loved one?

Even if you feel powerless to deal with AD's progression, there have been many studies on alternative therapies ranging from vitamin supplements to music and pet therapies that have helped some Alzheimer's disease patients.

Not all doctors are equally supportive of alternative therapies in general. But you may find that experimenting with recreational activities, healthy menus, mentally challenging puzzles, and social events will keep your loved one's agitation under control and give you a more positive mind-set.

This second doctor may suggest different treatments, including newer drugs and therapies that your primary care physician is unfamiliar with.

10. In your opinion, what is my/my loved one's prognosis after going through the treatment plan you've outlined?

Try to refrain from asking this question too early in the discussion. This way you can really listen to everything else this doctor has to say and make a well-informed decision about whether or not you like his treatment plan, personal style, and his potential to support you as the caregiver in the upcoming months.

Pay attention to how detailed and personalized his answer is to this question as another indication of the probable knowledge and quality of this doctor.

❯ The Magic Question

What advice would you give to your mother (sister, wife) to help her choose between the different recommendations/diagnosis/treatment options I've received?

If the first and second doctors disagree on the diagnosis or treatment plan, you may be confronted with a situation in which you have to choose between them without really knowing which one is better.

Rather than trying to be the Lone Ranger here and solve this

> **THE QUESTION DOCTOR SAYS:**
>
> Reduce the cost and time required for a second opinion by asking your first doctor to send copies of all tests results to the second-opinion doctor, if you choose not to have a "blind" second opinion. Take a friend or family member and a tape recorder to this office visit. That way you'll be able to listen and can compare notes and recordings later between the first and second doctors.

problem yourself, this Magic Question will put the second-opinion doctor's thinking cap on and engage him in helping you make the best decision. If needed, you can also go back to your first doctor and ask this same question and then compare answers.

Another strategy is to ask the two doctors to confer on your case and see if they can arrive at a mutual decision. You might also want to ask for a third opinion and then compare.

CONCLUSION

Why get a second opinion? The fundamental question when you are considering second opinions is really, "Why not?"

Asking for a second opinion is a frequent practice, growing more common, and some insurance plans even recommend it. Don't worry about hurting a doctor's feelings or insulting his intelligence by wanting a second opinion, even if he's your old favorite family doctor. The best doctors will actively support you. Often, patients choose to stay with their first doctor after seeking a second opinion from another doctor.

Alzheimer's disease is a frightening and complex disease. You deserve to have all the information and support you need to help you and your loved one deal with it. Seeking a second opinion may give you some peace of mind, knowing that you've done everything possible to ensure an accurate diagnosis.

THE 10 BEST RESOURCES

About.com. "Second Opinions: Why It's Important to Get a Second Opinion." http://lungdiseases.about.com/od/lungcancer/a/secondopinions.htm.

Alzheimer's Association. "Alzheimer's Disease Study: Communication Gaps Between Primary Care Physicians and Caregivers." www.alz.org/national/documents/report_communicationgap.pdf.

Alzheimer's Association. "Partnering with Your Doctor: A Guide for Persons with Memory Problems and Their Care Partners." www.alz.org/national/documents/brochure_partneringwithyourdoctor.pdf.

Cancer Research UK. "Seeing a Different Doctor for a Second Opinion." www.cancerhelp.org.uk/help/default.asp?page=20395.

Centers for Medicare and Medicaid Services. "Getting a Second Opinion Before Surgery." www.medicare.gov/Publications/Pubs/pdf/02173.pdf.

Eldercare Team. "Getting a Second Opinion." www.eldercareteam.com/resources/articles/secondopinion.htm.

Groopman, Jerome. "The Uncertainty of the Expert." In *How Doctors Think*. Boston: Houghton Mifflin, 2007.

Levine, Evan. *What Your Doctor Won't (or Can't) Tell You: The Failures of American Medicine—and How to Avoid Becoming a Statistic.* New York: Berkley, 2005.

Miller, Jim. "Savvy Senior: Second Opinion Can Buy Peace of Mind." *Charleston Gazette*, May 10, 2004, P2D.

U.S. Department of Health and Human Services, Agency for Healthcare Research and Quality. "Quick Tips—When Talking with Your Doctor." www.ahrq.gov/consumer/quicktips/doctalk.htm.

PART II:

Choosing Treatments

Discovering that you or your loved one has Alzheimer's disease is terribly confusing and upsetting. You suddenly find you must make important decisions about health care but it's hard to know all the facts or where to turn for advice. Most newly diagnosed Alzheimer's patients and their families describe feeling overwhelmed and panicked.

There are as many uniquely personal reactions to a diagnosis of Alzheimer's disease (AD) as there are uniquely different manifestations of the disease. Not everyone wants to do a lot of research or become a walking encyclopedia on AD. Yet others wouldn't have it any other way. Some people reach out to dozens of people for comfort and advice while others choose to keep their news private for as long as possible.

The 10 Best Questions in this section will help you to strengthen your decision-making muscles. Because Alzheimer's disease is not curable, you and your doctor will look for the best ways to prevent further cognitive decline with a combination of drugs, alternative therapies, and smart strategies for brain fitness. There are chapters on each of these key decision crossroads, along with the 10 Best Questions to help you avoid becoming a victim of scams for bogus alternative therapies and the 10 Best Questions to decide whether or not you want to participate in a clinical research trial. Knowing how you feel, sorting through your personal priorities, and learning about your treatment options will bring you a significant measure of comfort and self-confidence. A diagnosis of AD in its early stages or of mild cognitive impairment (MCI) is a window of opportunity for the person affected, since he can still actively participate in treatment decisions.

The Question Doctor sincerely hopes the following chapters and Best Questions on treatment choices will ease your journey. Your doctor may be an authority on medicine, but you are the world's foremost expert on yourself and your loved one.

CHAPTER 6: THE 10 BEST QUESTIONS
to Ask About Alzheimer's Drugs

The drug that heals our sorrows is forgetfulness.
—Appianus, second-century Greek historian

Alzheimer's is a slow disease that starts with mild memory loss and advances to severe brain damage and death. On average, Alzheimer's patients live from seven to ten years after a diagnosis, with some living up to twenty years.

Thousands of researchers across the world have devoted their entire professional lives to discovering drugs that can halt or reverse the effects of Alzheimer's disease. There are five drugs currently approved by the U.S. Food and Drug Administration for AD. Each of these drugs can only temporarily slow cognitive decline. There is no known treatment for Alzheimer's that either prevents or reverses the progression of brain cell death.

For treating cognitive symptoms, there are four drugs collectively known as **cholinesterase inhibitors**. These are usually prescribed for people with mild cognitive impairment (MCI) and early to moderate-stage Alzheimer's. A fifth drug, Namenda (memantine) is prescribed for the treatment of moderate to severe AD.

In addition to specific drugs for AD, other medications help to control behavioral and psychiatric symptoms, including agitation, outbursts, anxiety, depression, hallucinations, wandering, and sleeplessness. Treating these symptoms often makes AD patients more comfortable while easing their caregivers' burdens. Most AD patients are elderly and often need additional medications for prior medical conditions, such as heart disease or diabetes.

Pathologist and Alzheimer's disease expert Dr. Roger A. Brumback explains that the "blood brain barrier," or the natural barrier of brain blood vessels to the nerve cells that selectively allows nutrients and chemicals to pass through to the nerve cells, grows weaker with age. This process explains why the elderly are susceptible to overmedication. Dr. Brumback says, "There are many effects of medicines in older brains that you wouldn't see in a forty-year-old brain. Alzheimer's disease can be made tremendously worse by drug interactions that make the remaining healthy brain cells have to work harder."

The following Best Questions for your doctor are questions to be asked either by persons with MCI or early stage AD or their caregivers. Be sure to check with your insurance carrier and/or Medicare about payment coverage details.

THE QUESTION DOCTOR SAYS:

Consider taking a tape recorder or a notepad with you for this office visit. Many people are intimidated by discussions about complex drugs with long, unpronounceable names. You can listen to the tape later or review your notes without the additional pressure of being face to face with the doctor.

〉〉〉THE 10 BEST QUESTIONS
to Ask About Alzheimer's Drugs

1. **What drugs are available to me/my loved one? Please explain how these drugs work.**

There are four drugs prescribed for Alzheimer's called "cholinesterase inhibitors":

1. Donepezil (Aricept)
2. Galantamine (Razadyne, previously known as Reminyl)

3. Rivastigmine (Exelon)
4. Tacrine (Cognex, limited availability)

Each of these drugs is thought to boost the levels of the neurotransmitter acetylcholine, a chemical messenger in the brain, and slow the body's normal process that breaks down acetylcholine.

The cholinesterase inhibitors are prescribed mainly for early stage AD and MCI, although Aricept is also used for moderate to severe AD. These drugs delay cognitive symptoms for a limited time. Scientists don't fully understand yet exactly why these drugs work.

A fifth drug, Namenda (memantine) is prescribed for treating moderate to severe AD. Researchers believe Namenda works by regulating glutamate, another important brain chemical that may lead to the death of brain cells when it's produced in excessive amounts. Taking Namenda allows some patients to maintain their daily functions, such as continence, longer.

2. What percentage of improvement can I reasonably expect from this drug?

As you weigh the potential risks and benefits of taking any drug, hearing about the positive effects as a number may help clarify the facts. Ask your doctor to talk in specific terms, such as the average percentage of improvement or the average length of time patients with AD similar to yours can live reduced-symptom lives with this drug.

No doctor can predict with absolute certainty how well an AD medication will halt cognitive decline, but this discussion will help you establish realistic expectations. Be sure to ask your doctor to explain the potential benefits for you personally and not just national averages or the "average case."

This question also works for the behavioral drugs. Again, you may hear only a range of numbers rather than an exact estimate for improvement.

3. How will you know if this drug is working well?

It's equally important to understand the details of how your doctor plans to assess and monitor a proposed drug's effectiveness over time.

As AD progresses, the patient is less capable of communicating with either the doctor or the caregiver. To further complicate matters, every AD patient has a slightly different disease progression, which makes standard assessments of cognitive drugs more difficult. The effectiveness of behavioral drugs is more readily apparent, since changes in behavior are more visual and obvious than changes in thinking and mental function.

4. What short-term side effects are possible? Long-term side effects? Any side effects that may not go away?

The AD drugs' most common side effects include nausea, vomiting, loss of appetite, and a change in bowel habits such as constipation or an increased frequency of bowel movements. Cognex may also cause liver damage so it has limited availability. You may be drug-sensitive or experience drug interactions with your other prescription medications, vitamins, or herbal supplements. Older people in general don't eliminate drugs as quickly from their systems as younger people do, which can cause drugs to build up to toxic levels.

Be sure your doctor addresses this question for your specific case and not just with data from clinical trials or general studies. Also be sure to ask about potential long-term or permanent side effects, questions few people think to ask.

5. How will you (the doctor) help me to manage side effects?

This question will help you to learn more about side effects and if there are ways to lessen their impact on your health. For example, if you experience stomach upset, which is common with the cholinesterase inhibitors, there may be simple over-the-counter remedies or another prescription that will help control this problem.

6. What can I do to minimize the side effects and stay healthy?

Asking this question will help you feel like you are more in control of your own health. This question also implies that you and your doctor are a team, with both of you actively involved in your care and well-being.

Inquire how alternative treatments, diet, and exercise might affect this drug's effectiveness. See chapter 7 for more on living a healthy lifestyle.

7. What, if any, restrictions will there be on my normal activities while taking this drug?

Be sure you understand if there are prohibitions on any foods, other drugs, alcohol use, or any additional considerations you should know in advance. This is especially true if you still live a normal and active lifestyle, including travel, work, and outdoor activities.

8. How long will I be taking this drug before you are able to evaluate the drug's effectiveness?

This Best Question is suggested by the national Alzheimer's Association. The doctor's answer will help you be realistic about anticipated gains and give you more insights into how your doctor plans to monitor this drug over time.

9. What symptoms or changes in my mental or physical health are serious enough for me (or my caregiver) to call you?

Find out the specifics of what drug-related changes you should watch for at home. You shouldn't have to guess about whether or not a phone call to your doctor is necessary. Many caregivers hesitate to call their doctors for fear of "bothering" the doctor or over-reacting to new symptoms. Let your doctor's response guide you in making better-informed decisions.

10. What is my overall treatment plan?

In addition to discussing specific drugs, you'll be smart to find out the big picture for your long-term care and treatment. Be sure your doctor's plan includes both AD medications and behavioral and psychiatric treatments as well.

Your doctor will probably start you at a low dosage to see how well you tolerate the drug and to monitor side effects. He may gradually increase the dosage, but you may start having more side effects. Because Namenda works differently than the cholinesterase inhibitors, it can be prescribed with them for combination therapy.

Find out if any proposed treatment options will interfere with your other medications. You also need to understand any medical concerns with switching or stopping drugs. Because of their similarities, switching among the cholinesterase inhibitors will probably not result in significantly different results, although you may tolerate one drug better than the others.

Finally, get a sense from your doctor at what stage it will be appropriate for you to no longer receive this drug or other treatments. As AD progresses, the cholinesterase inhibitors lose their effectiveness because there are fewer and fewer existing brain cells to respond to the drug.

❯ The Magic Question

What happens if I choose not to take any drugs to treat my Alzheimer's? How clear-cut is my case for taking the drug(s) you are recommending?

Seniors are the largest consumers of the $200 billion per year we spend on prescription drugs in America. Drug companies spend enormous amounts of money and effort to convince doctors and AD patients that their products are a worthy investment. With a diagnosis as frightening as Alzheimer's, you may not stop to consider, "What exactly am I putting in my body?" "Is it worth it?" "Is this drug a good value for my money?"

This Magic Question was a Best Question for your primary care physician at the time of your initial diagnosis. It's here again because it's so important (and so often overlooked) to explore this option with a specialist in Alzheimer's disease.

Rather than automatically assuming your best bet is to take drugs, ask now if doing nothing may be a viable option. The answer depends on many variables, such as your age, other medical conditions or prescriptions, financial situation, and living and care arrangements. All AD drugs only slow the disease; none can permanently stop or reverse it. Behavioral drugs may not yet be necessary or may be ill-advised in your case. These drugs are expensive. You may have limited insurance coverage or live on a fixed income.

CONCLUSION

Use your doctor's advice and answers to make a better-informed decision about treatment. If you are still unsure what to do, ask your doctor this follow-up question: "If you were making this decision for your parent or loved one with AD, what would you do?"

Consider your personal priorities and financial situation as you ask *yourself* these two follow-up questions: "Are these drugs cost effective for me?" "Will they improve the quality of life for me and my caregiver?"

Everyone's disease and situations are different, so there is no single right or wrong answer. Some people are happy for any slight improvement, while others dismiss small improvements as insufficient to justify the costs or hassle. Your quality of life issues are an important consideration as you evaluate what's best for you and your family.

THE 10 BEST RESOURCES

Alzheimer's Association. "FDA-Approved Treatments for Alzheimer's." www.alz.org/national/documents/topicsheet_treatments.pdf.

Alzheimer's Association. "Taking Medications Safely." http://www.alz .org/national/documents/topicsheet_medsafety.pdf.

Alzheimer's Association. "Standard Treatments." www.alz.org/alzheimers_ disease_standard_prescriptions.asp.

Alzheimer's Disease Education and Referral Center. "Alzheimer's Disease Medications Fact Sheet." www.nia.nih.gov/Alzheimers/Publications/medi cationsfs.htm.

Food and Drug Administration. "Drug Information Pathfinder." www .fda.gov/cder/offices/DDI/pathfinder.htm.

Hurley, Dan. "Dementia Drugs Demystified: What to Expect—and Not to Expect—from Alzheimer's Medications." *Neurology Now.* September/ October 2006, 32–33. Issue archive at www.neurologynow.com.

Mayo Clinic. "Alzheimer's Drugs Slow Progression of Disease." www .mayoclinic.com/health/alzheimers/AZ00015.

Medicare. "Medicare Prescription Drug Plan Finder." www.medicare.gov/ MPDPF.

MedlinePlus. "Drugs, Supplements, and Herbal Information." Database searchable by drug name. www.nlm.nih.gov/medlineplus/druginformation.html.

MetLife. "Medications and the Older Adult." www.metlife.com/FileAssets/MMI/MMISYCMedications.pdf.

CHAPTER 7: THE 10 BEST QUESTIONS
for Brain Fitness

> Old age is the most unexpected of all the things that
> can happen to a man.
>
> —Leon Trotsky

There is a wide choice of alternative treatments (also called **complementary treatments** or **integrated medicine**) that can temporarily improve the quality of life for you and your loved one, especially with a MCI or early stage Alzheimer's diagnosis. In fact, in the absence of any medications that are indisputably effective, many AD experts advocate lifestyle changes and alternative treatments as the best hope for slowing the disease's progression.

Dr. Gary Small, director of UCLA's Memory and Aging Center and author of *The Memory Bible*, says, "By the time a patient develops Alzheimer's disease, the damage is done and likely irreversible. In the absence of a cure, our best shot at beating Alzheimer's lies in targeting mild forgetfulness with lifestyle changes."

Lifestyle changes focus on improving diet and exercise habits, using promising vitamins and supplements, and undertaking challenging mental activities to keep the brain going for as long as possible. Alternative treatments include gardening, keeping a pet, attending social events, acupuncture, aromatherapy, massage, music, and art therapies, among others.

Even for moderate- and late-stage Alzheimer's patients, there are many simple tasks that the person can do. Caregiver Elaine Marshall in Leesburg, Virginia, says, "It takes my mother hours to fold a basket of laundry that I could do in five minutes. But I think it's important to give her a sense of purpose and a task she can still do. She feels like she is still contributing to the family, which is priceless."

Be sure to ask your doctor for his advice before you or your loved one takes any dietary supplements, embarks on an exercise plan, or goes on a serious weight-loss diet. You want your doctor's blessing that your alternative treatment will not interfere with prescription medications or dangerously aggravate another medical condition, such as heart trouble or diabetes.

These following Best Questions are for persons with MCI or early stage dementia to ask themselves, but they can easily be adjusted to work equally well for the caregiver who is contemplating alternative treatments for his loved one. You can also take them to your doctor's office and use them as the basis of a discussion with her about developing a customized alternative treatment plan for you or your loved one.

〉〉〉THE 10 BEST QUESTIONS
for Brain Fitness

1. What can I do to eat better and maintain a healthy weight?

Adopt a healthy diet of brain-protective foods. Good nutrition and diligent weight management are constantly cited as especially necessary for people with Alzheimer's. The best nutritional advice includes to "eat the rainbow" of varied, colorful vegetables and fruits to ensure you're getting the full range of disease-fighting phytochemicals (plant compounds) and antioxidants.

Other dietary goals are to eat well-balanced meals, whole grains, and the mono- and polyunsaturated fats in nuts, seeds, and some vegetable oils. There is growing evidence that the omega-3 fatty acids found in fish such as salmon, sardines, tuna, and trout are linked to a lower risk of Alzheimer's.

Weight management is a struggle for more than two-thirds of

all adult Americans. A long-term study found that those who were obese in middle age were twice as likely to develop dementia later in life.

Overweight early stage AD patients can renew their efforts to shed pounds by making a commitment, setting realistic goals, and getting emotional support. For late-stage AD patients, the challenge is often the opposite—to avoid losing weight as their appetites decline or they simply forget to eat regular meals. Good nutrition equals good blood flow and brain health.

2. How can I make exercise a natural part of my daily routine?

Burning more calories and working the heart and lungs harder will lengthen and improve your quality of life as you age. Anything that gets your heart rate up counts, like walking, climbing stairs, or playing ball with your grandchildren, ideally to add up to about thirty minutes most days of the week.

The biggest challenge for many people in trying to maintain an exercise routine is being consistent and exercising every day. If this sounds familiar, do something to really encourage yourself, such as taking a walk at the same time each morning or walking with a friend, until it becomes a habit as ingrained as brushing your teeth every day.

3. Which supplements, herbs, and vitamins can I take for treating Alzheimer's?

Preliminary research studies suggest there are positive benefits from certain vitamins, herbal remedies, and dietary supplements if you have AD. The following are commonly cited as having possible benefits for AD patients.

- Omega-3 fatty acids (in natural and supplement forms)
- Vitamins B_{12}, B_6, and B_9 (folic acid), and vitamins C, D, and E

- Herbs (*Ginkgo biloba*, ginseng, and others)
- Huperzine A (Chinese medicinal extract with properties similar to cholinesterase inhibitors)

However, none of these has yet proved to be a clear winner. Each needs further research to prove its benefits conclusively and to identify possible side effects. As a result, most of these products aren't regulated or federally controlled for purity and safety, which can put consumers at serious risk. See chapter 8 on spotting scams.

4. Where can I find mentally challenging activities? How can I stay curious about the world around me?

Many experts believe in the "use it or lose it" theory when it comes to brain functioning. A love of lifelong learning, "mental aerobics," and the active pursuit of new interests (yes, even for Alzheimer's patients) are key components to slowing down mental decline. Being curious is a vital touchstone to staying engaged in the world around you, from reading the daily news to caring about someone else's experiences.

There are many special Alzheimer activity books to help you retain your reading and communication skills for early stage independent use or later to share and reminisce with a caregiver. You can challenge your brain with crossword puzzles, playing bridge or chess, charades, and other puzzles or games you enjoy.

Music's effect on memory and emotions is the subject of a fast-growing research field. The American Music Therapy Association (www.musictherapy.org) claims that even people with advanced AD can recall old favorite songs and benefit from musical expression. Similarly, art therapy keeps open your creative and nonverbal communication outlets.

Other enjoyable and mentally stimulating activities include field trips, gardening and horticulture, and educational travel

> **THE QUESTION DOCTOR SAYS:**
>
> Asking questions is good brain food, too! The curiosity behind your questions is a high-order cognitive skill that leads to more exploring, learning, and imagining, all part of a healthy brain diet. Move over, curious kitty, and keep those questions coming.

through senior programs such as Elderhostel, which has thousands of national and international programs.

Maybe you don't want to traipse with Elderhostel to China and stay in a hotel without a Western-style bathroom. If so, just be smart about your small choices, too. Watch an episode of the mentally challenging television quiz show *Jeopardy* tonight instead of another rerun of *Friends*.

5. How can I live a more toxin-free life?

There is growing evidence that many of the chemicals and toxins in our everyday lives are potential killers. These include lead and household chemicals, chemicals in highly processed foods, and the plastics used for water or soda bottles. Aluminum in the diet has been linked to Alzheimer's for years, although its definite connection is still undetermined.

Buying and preparing foods yourself, especially fresh produce and meats, is a key way to know and control what goes into your body. If you are concerned, consider buying organic foods. One mantra, "Eat less, pay more," summarizes the advantages of eating controlled quantities of better-quality food (such as fresh fruits and vegetables) instead of less costly potato chips.

Other obvious sources of toxins are smoking (including second-hand smoke), street drugs, and overindulgence in alcohol.

6. What can I do to reduce the stress in my life?

Chill out. There's a vast amount of research that says that excessive stress can result in mental confusion, heart disease, and reduced immunity. Seek stress-reduction techniques like yoga, meditation, laughter, talking about feelings, and physical exercise. Ironically, a common cause of stress is worrying about memory performance or a family history of AD.

Job stress can be especially tough on newly diagnosed AD patients who feel torn between continuing their work and worry about declining mental abilities. Consider your retirement options or part-time employment.

There are also nontraditional ways of reducing stress in your life, such as pet therapy. You may be surprised at the stress-busting effects of caring for a pet now or later in a nursing home. The Delta Society offers special programs (www.deltasociety.org). The effects of aromatherapy (use of mood-enhancing oils) and acupuncture (therapeutic use of small needles) on stress are still being explored. Music, massage, and art therapies all reduce stress, too.

7. Am I sleeping well and long enough? If not, what can I do about it?

A good night's sleep for most people means seven to eight hours a night. Getting enough sleep is a staple tip for people looking to live longer and boost their mental capacities, according to the newest research. If you don't snooze, you lose.

Sleep disturbances become increasingly common with more advanced AD stages. More nighttime restlessness and agitation make it harder to fall and stay asleep, upsetting the caregiver's sleep, too.

Check with your doctor about advice or medication if you are currently unable to sleep well. A more active lifestyle and better diet may also improve your sleep during early stage AD.

8. How can I maintain my social connections?

Being social can keep the blues away. Life is more fun when it's shared with friends and family members. Many studies have concluded that you can maintain your brain by maintaining your personal relationships.

If you live alone with MCI or early stage AD, pay special attention to keeping connected to others as a way to jog your brain. Senior centers and activities, adult day care, family reunions, and friendly get-togethers are all occasions that keep the brain cells charged and your neurons firing.

9. What cause or purpose inspires me and is worth my time and energy to pursue actively?

Find a cause such as global warming, volunteer work, or a neighborhood eyesore to improve—whatever matters to you.

Author and senior Alzheimer's researcher Dr. Peter Whitehouse says, "Older people need a sense of purpose and community. Being engaged is a way of creating your own legacy. This focus is more important than medications."

There are innovative programs that pair senior citizens in adult day care with children in child care for mutual stimulation, reading, and bonding. Some people find their purpose in their spirituality, religious beliefs, or by serving in their church or synagogue. There's no right or wrong cause as long as it's important to you.

10. How can I protect my head from injuries?

Researchers still aren't clear on the possible relationship between previous head injuries and the onset or worsening of AD symptoms, but a nasty bump on the head sure can't help anything either. Older people need to protect themselves from falls and do head-smart things like wear their seatbelts or bicycle helmets.

❯ The Magic Question

What activities in the past gave me the greatest pleasure? How can I adapt these activities to my current situation of living with Alzheimer's?

Reassess and reconnect with your lifelong pleasures and skills. Maybe you were always handy with a hammer or a mechanic's wrench. Perhaps raising beefsteak tomatoes, tinkering with old cars, or knitting mohair sweaters was your thing.

Reflect on doing that special interest or skill again within your current limitations and while taking appropriate safety precautions. Just realize that your days of handling a chain saw or blowtorch are probably over.

A fun example is the Australian group Blokes with Sheds (www.ibys.org/blokes_and_sheds.html). Elderly men with dementia build sheds in a meaningful version of a giant jigsaw puzzle. Advanced AD patients can sort the screws, nails, and bolts, although they must be supervised so no one tries to swallow the hammer! See Alzheimer's Australia for more information (www.alzheimers.org.au/upload/sheds.pdf).

CONCLUSION

There are no known cures and no one knows for sure what causes Alzheimer's disease. The scientific debate on the value of alternative treatments, diet, exercise, and other lifestyle issues continue as new research studies produce often conflicting results.

Author and AD expert Daniel Kuhn says, "Alternative medicine is a largely ignored piece of the Alzheimer's puzzle . . . There are lots of things that can be done to improve the quality of life apart from medical treatments."

The suggestions here are science's current best bets in helping you or your loved one to manage the gradual decline of brain function. Instead of thinking fitness from the neck down, it's time to pay attention to jogging your brain, too.

THE 10 BEST RESOURCES

Alzheimer's Association. "Inside the Brain: An Interactive Tour." www
.alz.org/alzheimers_disease_4719.asp.

Bazan-Salazar, Emilia C. *Alzheimer's Activities that Stimulate the Mind.*
New York: McGraw-Hill, 2005.

Bell, Virginia, and David Troxel, Tonya M. Cox, and Robin Hamon. *The Best Friends Book of Alzheimer's Activities,* vol. 2. Baltimore, Md.: Health Professions Press, 2007.

Dowling, James R. *Keeping Busy: A Handbook of Activities for Persons with Dementia.* Baltimore, Md.: The Johns Hopkins University Press, 1995.

Goldman, Robert, and Lisa Berger. *Brain Fitness.* New York: Doubleday, 1999.

Kuhn, Daniel. "Keeping a Person with AD Active and Healthy." in *Alzheimer's Early Stages: First Steps for Family, Friends and Caregivers.* Alameda, Calif.: Hunter House Publishers, 2003.

McKhann, Guy M., and Marilyn Albert. *Keep Your Brain Young: The Complete Guide to Physical and Emotional Health and Longevity.* Hoboken, N.J.: John Wiley and Sons, 2002.

Medina, John. *Brain Rules: 12 Principles for Surviving and Thriving at Work, Home, and School.* Seattle, Wash.: Pear Press, 2008.

Small, Gary. *The Memory Bible: An Innovative Strategy for Keeping Your Brain Young.* New York: Hyperion, 2003.

Wikipedia. "Brain Fitness." www.en.wikipedia.org/wiki/Brain_fitness.

CHAPTER 8: THE 10 BEST QUESTIONS

to Avoid Alternative Treatment Scams

A quack doctor can kill you without a knife.

—Chinese proverb

You may not realize it, but you are exceedingly vulnerable to losing a wad of money to a con artist specializing in bogus alternative Alzheimer's treatments. The U.S. Department of Health and Human Services, the Federal Trade Commission, and the Food and Drug Administration all warn that because AD is such a devastating disease with no clearly superior treatments, desperate patients and their families can be easily tempted to try unproven, unscientific, and sometimes dangerous cures.

You are like a dinner bell to con artists promoting their snake oil supplements, herbs, and memory-enhancing systems. These unscrupulous con artists who prey on AD patients, caregivers, and elderly people in general know how to take advantage of your needs, emotions, and fears. Even if you think you are too savvy to get scammed, the many slick Web sites with impressive-sounding medical lingo, big promises, and endless testimonials from "happily cured" AD patients might still be intriguing.

This next set of 10 Best Questions will help you to make more objective decisions when you are assessing the claims of an alternative treatment promotion or Web site. Some alternative treatments are unpleasant, like drinking raw liver juice, or downright dangerous, like taking megadoses of vitamins. Hold the liver juice and read the following Best Questions instead.

THE QUESTION DOCTOR SAYS:

The following Best Questions are aimed at Web sites claiming to provide alternative Alzheimer's treatments. You can easily adjust the questions to use while you are reviewing mail advertisements, dealing with a telephone sales call, or talking to salesmen face to face about their alternative products for treating AD.

>>> THE 10 BEST QUESTIONS
to Avoid Alternative Treatment Scams

1. Who's behind this claim or alternative therapy?

Any Web site or company offering medical therapies should make it easy to learn who is responsible and should provide their medical credentials. Even if someone has important sounding initials after his name, question where he works, his training, and search his name on the Internet. Expect to see a history of his publications in professional medical journals.

Run the other way as fast as you can if no one is home at this Web site or the company, or if the principals don't have impressive professional histories in memory-related areas.

As Dr. Stephen Barrett, founder of the consumer watchdog Web site Quackwatch, warns, "Don't let desperation cloud your judgment."

2. Are the people offering the alternative therapies also the same people who are selling them?

The funding sources behind this Web site should be clearly explained. Information from a neutral or disinterested third party is usually more reliable than those from someone who benefits personally from product sales. There's a certain measure of consumer security in Web sites that indicate a nonprofit status.

3. Is this therapy a cure, remission, or healing offer?

Alternative therapies include high-dose vitamin supplements, diets, herbal remedies, gadgets, and dietary practices like detoxification. Not all are bad for you or bogus, but some are potentially harmful. Avoid Web sites with flowery medical jargon, claims to cure Alzheimer's (impossible), and multiple ads on the Web site, especially ones that offer money-back guarantees or free trial supplements.

The Alzheimer's Association cites its concerns about alternative AD drugs:

- Unknown effectiveness or safety
- Unknown purity
- No monitoring of bad reactions
- Dietary supplements can interfere with prescription drugs

These scammers are very good at fooling folks, even extremely well-educated people. Read these Web sites carefully several times or ask for a trusted friend's opinion.

4. Does the Web site or company have a seal of credibility?

If the Web site or company does not have an approval or accreditation seal, that doesn't automatically make it a bogus organization but a seal of credibility provides you with extra assurances about a company's professionalism. Check with Health on the Net (www .hon.ch) and URAC (formerly the Utilization Review Accreditation Council, www.urac.org) to verify seals.

5. Is this alternative therapy offered as a "miracle" cure?

Look out for phrases like "scientific breakthrough," "miraculous cure," "secret ingredient," or "ancient remedy." Don't believe claims that say they are credible because they have endured for decades or centuries or have many "testimonials" claiming phenomenal success rates. Look out for extravagant claims using words like "always" or "never."

For example, quacks sell diet supplements by first stating that all Americans are poorly nourished and all disease, including AD, stems from bad eating habits. Their follow-up statement, of course, is that the only solution is their own "miracle" megadoses of a vitamin or herb.

6. Are any prior studies offered as scientific evidence, or are there only anecdotal stories and personal testimonials to back up the claimed benefits of this alternative therapy?

You want specific scientific evidence including measurable results in hard, cold numbers, not that it tasted good and Sam with advanced AD could suddenly memorize the Gettysburg Address afterward.

7. What other documentation is given to support the Web site's or company's claims?

Look for more information sources and references, especially in established medical journals, not e-magazines or blogs. Be wary of listings that are old or stopped being updated more than a year ago.

8. Does this alternative therapy or company claim to have exclusive rights to the treatments offered?

Real Alzheimer's treatments have well-documented studies with hundreds or thousands of patients. Fake treatments are available from only one doctor, clinic, or Web site. It doesn't make sense there would be a monopoly on new products or treatments as good as these.

9. Has any conventional medical organization endorsed this product or treatment?

Endorsements by trusted names in medical science and neurology are a good sign. In contrast, scammers emphasize that others—usually highly respected doctors or "the establishment"—are trying to suppress the distribution of their products.

10. Is personal information or money requested up front?

Avoid Web sites that won't give you the facts about their products until you've created an account with them, revealing your name, e-mail address, credit card number, Medicare details, or other personal information. Other red flags are requests for money up front or the offering of a perpetual discount, like "40 percent off."

❯ The Magic Question

If a medical breakthrough really had occurred for Alzheimer's disease, would the news be announced first in an ad?

The credit for this commonsense Magic Question belongs to the Federal Trade Commission, the federal government's watchdog organization. The con artists' claim of "exclusive rights" is the ultimate tip-off that you're dealing with bogus treatments.

CONCLUSION

It's important to be proactive in seeking alternative treatments for Alzheimer's. At the same time, you don't want to be the next victim of a fake treatment that could potentially endanger your loved one's health and well-being—and cost you a bundle for nothing.

Many of these bogus health companies and products are run by people who understand perfectly—maybe better than you—your vulnerabilities in this situation. If someone wants to sell you unproven supplements, magic herbs, a cure for MCI, or a miracle brain exerciser, now you know what to ask them first. If you are still unsure, ask your doctor to verify a product's benefits and safety before purchasing it.

THE 10 BEST RESOURCES

Administration on Aging. "Consumer Protection Tips." www.aoa.gov/smp/consprof/consprof_resources_tips.asp.

Barrett, Stephen, and Victor Herbert. "Twenty-Five Ways to Spot Quacks and Vitamin Pushers." www.quackwatch.com/01QuackeryRelatedTopics/spotquack.html.

Federal Citizen Information Center. "State, County, and City Government Consumer Protection Offices." www.consumeraction.gov/state.shtml.

Federal Trade Commission. "Virtual 'Treatments' Can Be Real-World Deceptions." www.ftc.gov/bcp/conline/pubs/alerts/mrclalrt.shtm.

Food and Drug Administration. "2008 Safety Alerts for Drugs, Biologics, Medical Devices, and Dietary Supplements." www.fda.gov/medwatch/safety/2008/safety08.htm.

Food and Drug Administration. "Buying Prescription Medicine Online: A Consumer Safety Guide." www.fda.gov/cder/consumerinfo/buyOnlineGuide_text.htm.

Health on the Net Foundation. "HONcode Site Evaluation Form." www.hon.ch/HONcode/HONcode_check.html.

National Institute on Aging. "Health Quackery: Spotting Health Scams." www.nia.nih.gov/HealthInformation/Publications/quackery.htm.

National Institute on Aging. "Online Health Information: Can You Trust It?" www.nia.nih.gov/HealthInformation/Publications/onlinehealth.htm.

URAC. "Consumer Resource Center." www.urac.org/consumers/resources.

Before Participating in a Clinical Trial

> Today, only a small percentage of consumers are aware
> of clinical trials as a health care option, both from a
> standpoint of receiving a high level of care and in helping
> develop the latest products to treat debilitating or life-
> threatening diseases.
>
> —Dr. C. Everett Koop, former U.S. Surgeon General,
> during a 2006 interview with the author

A **clinical trial** is a research program conducted with patients to evaluate a new medical treatment, drug, or device. The purpose of a clinical trial for Alzheimer's disease
is to try to determine what causes this disease, find new cures, or
clarify what lifestyle choices, such as diet, exercise, or certain supplemental vitamins, may be curative measures.

Clinical trials (also called "clinical studies") make it possible to
apply the latest scientific and technological advances to patient
care. During an Alzheimer's clinical trial, researchers, usually doctors, test a drug or treatment with the hopes that the experiment
will relieve AD symptoms, delay the onset of advanced disease, or
reduce the risk of an early death.

It's important that AD patients and their families understand
that because Alzheimer's disease is so complex, it's not likely that a
single drug or cure will be discovered through any one given clinical trial. If you are interested in being involved with a clinical trial,
just be realistic about the unlikelihood that a miracle cure will be
found. Every study and person involved matters, but realistically,
scientific progress is usually gained by small steps forward in many
clinical studies, not giant leaps or quick miracle drugs.

On the positive side, according to the Alzheimer's Association, research indicates that people who are involved in clinical studies do somewhat better than others at a similar stage of their disease, regardless of the experiment's outcome. From a patient's perspective, the other benefits of participating in a clinical trial include:

- Increased patient monitoring, more surveillance by a medical team, and generally a higher standard of AD care than normally available
- Health care benefits, such as free genetic tests for family members
- Long-term information and better preventive care for family members who may be at risk for AD too
- The opportunity to make a personal contribution in the fight against this terrible disease

In 2004, more than 17 million people inquired about participating in clinical trials in the United States, and more than 2 million people volunteered for industry- and government-sponsored studies. More than eighty thousand clinical trials (all diseases) are conducted in the United States annually. The growing number of participants indicates a trend toward patients' increasing receptivity for clinical trials as one of their medical options.

However, even though the majority of clinical trials are safe and effective, there are risks for volunteers. According to a 2002 study by CenterWatch, a Boston-based publisher of clinical trial information, the majority of people (70 percent) who enter clinical trials do so without knowing what questions to ask. This problem is further complicated for AD clinical trials when the patient's disease has progressed beyond the point that he can be fully aware of the informed consent process and the trial's details.

Another CenterWatch analysis of Food and Drug Administration data found that one in thirty volunteers typically experiences a serious side effect, and one in ten thousand dies as a result of effects of a study drug. Many people reported that they didn't fully understand the risks of study participation, and 10 percent of volunteers admitted they didn't even look at the informed consent form before signing it.

In 2007, there were more than 150 clinical studies on Alzheimer's disease that actively recruited participants, both with and without AD or related memory loss. To learn more about AD studies, see the Alzheimer's Disease Clinical Trials Database, a joint project of the U.S. Food and Drug Administration and the National Institute on Aging (NIA). The database is maintained by NIA's Alzheimer's Disease Education and Referral Center (ADEAR). To search the database for current trials, new trials, and trials making headlines, go to the ADEAR Web site (www.alzheimers.org/clinicaltrials/search.asp) or the Alzheimer's Association's Web site (www.alz.org/alzheimers_disease_clinical_studies.asp).

This chapter has two lists of 10 Best Questions. One list of Best Questions covers what to ask your doctor for more information about clinical trials. The other list of Best Questions are the ones to ask *yourself* in order to decide if participating in a clinical trial is right for you or your loved one.

Keep in mind that if you are considering a clinical trial, you may need to decide soon after diagnosis and before other treatments begin. Talk with your doctor about this point and ask him any other questions you have. The person with AD who is interested in clinical trials may want to include a statement to this effect in his or her advance directives (see chapter 24). Getting involved with AD research is a big step. You want to be fully informed and understand exactly what you're getting into ahead of time.

>>> THE 10 BEST QUESTIONS
to Ask Your Doctor Before Participating in a Clinical Trial

1. How will this trial help me personally?

Keep this conversation at the personal level—the benefits for you personally—rather than generic or statistical facts. Your bottom-line question is, "What's in it for me and my loved one?" Be sure you understand your doctor's comparison of your routine treatment plan versus the treatments you'd receive as a participant in a clinical trial.

Everyone's AD progression has its own unique characteristics, and different people respond differently to various drugs and treatments. One of the biggest possible drawbacks is the risk that you may be randomly assigned a **placebo drug,** which is an inactive, look-alike treatment. The people getting the placebo are the **control group,** which helps the scientists to factor out some people's favorable reaction to a new drug just because they believe it's working.

A placebo-controlled experiment helps the researchers know for sure that a new drug or treatment is the real reason for any positive health gains, not because people were hoping for the best. When neither the researchers nor the participants know which group is getting the experimental drug, this is called a **double-blind trial.** In most cases, the placebo group can receive the experimental drug after the trial ends if researchers find it effective.

This effort to prevent research bias can mean that the AD person is not receiving helpful drugs if she is part of the placebo group. According to the Alzheimer's Association, most trials have a built-in safety monitoring committee to step in if there are serious complications during the trial. But the fact still remains that some portion of the trial's participants will not receive the promising new drug or treatment.

2. What are the researchers hoping to learn from this study? What phase is this trial in?

Clinical trials are developed for different reasons. Some study the effectiveness of certain drugs, others study which doses are safe, and yet others look for ways of preventing Alzheimer's disease. Know the purpose of the study prior to signing on.

A key follow-up question is, "What phase is this trial?" Clinical trials are usually conducted in a series of steps of human testing, called Phase I, Phase II, Phase III, and Phase IV trials. **Preclinical studies** are studies conducted in the laboratory or with experimental animals to establish a scientific basis for the safety and potential benefits from experiments with human subjects.

Phase I trials are the first stage and usually enroll fewer than one hundred volunteers in limited locations. The primary purposes of Phase I trials are to assess drug safety, side effects, and risks.

Phase II trials study the effectiveness of a new drug or treatment in volunteers who have the condition being studied. A few hundred volunteers help researchers to establish a drug's effectiveness at different doses. The goal of Phase II trials is to establish that a new treatment substantially benefits at least 20 percent of patients who receive the drug.

Phase III trials provide hard, statistical evidence about whether a drug prolongs survival or improves quality of life and use several hundred or sometimes thousands of volunteers. These trials provide the main evidence the FDA will consider in making its decision on whether or not to approve a new drug.

Phase IV trials further evaluate the long-term safety and effectiveness of a drug and usually take place after a drug has been approved for standard use. Again, large numbers of volunteers are used, and their health is monitored to assess long-term drug safety and effectiveness.

3. Who is sponsoring this trial? Describe this trial's prior history and measurable outcomes.

This is an important question because it will help you understand more about the researchers' motives. The gold standard in clinical trials is sponsorship by a highly respected group such as the National Institutes of Health (NIH) or the National Institute on Aging (NIA). Drug companies can also offer solid and ethical trials. By understanding the trial's sponsors, you'll start to have clues into their possible biases. See The Magic Question at the end of the chapter, which provides more information on this topic.

Learn everything you can about the study's previous history. Some of this will be determined by what phase this particular clinical trial is in. Ask about the previous results, success rates, and the number of people involved. Get the details on how the study is being conducted and what specifically is asked of participants.

Ask the "who, what, when, where, and why" questions to prompt a full explanation from your doctor. Find out if you'll be required to switch doctors or Alzheimer's care centers. Another important consideration is stability. You don't necessarily want to be seen by a series of rotating doctors, each one being another "get acquainted" chore for you.

4. What are the possible risks and complications, both short term and long term, in my/our case?

Make sure the focus of this answer is about you and your loved one, rather than general statistics, which mean less to you personally. Be sure your doctor tells you as much as is known about possible long-term residual effects from taking an experimental drug or having a certain treatment.

Other potential risks include:

- The possibility that this experimental drug isn't as good as the current standard treatments
- The experimental drug may not work for you/your loved one personally
- Your health insurance carrier may not cover all study costs
- Some trials are time consuming or disruptive to daily routines, which may already be burdened by constant caregiving chores, and upsetting to Alzheimer patients

A really smart follow-up question in this discussion is, "What *don't* we know yet about this new drug or treatment?" This question will encourage your doctor to reveal candidly any design flaws and possible side effects. It's quite possible that there are many unknowns—that's the experimental nature of clinical trials. Or your doctor may not be fully informed about a particular trial. If so, ask for concrete guidance and specific information resources.

5. What safety measures are built into this study?

You want to understand how this study maximizes your potential benefits while minimizing potential harm. Your doctor's answer to this question should include detailed information about how patient safety will be monitored and a description of patient safeguards.

Ask, "Has this study been approved by an **institutional review board** (ethical panels made up of doctors and other medical experts who work with large hospitals or universities and the Food and Drug Administration)?" and "Did the review board that approved this trial have any ethical concerns with the trial?" Another key safety measure is to be sure that you/your loved one can quit the trial at any time without consequences. Also ask about how your personal and medical information will be protected from identify theft or other unauthorized disclosures.

6. How long does this trial last? Where is it being conducted?

The length of clinical trials varies greatly, as does the amount of time required of you on a daily, weekly, or monthly basis. Sometimes trials involve one day or one blood draw. Often, especially in drug trials, the trial will last for several months or even years. Know the expected duration of your trial before signing on. Be sure to find out the total time the trial will last (in months or years). Then ask, "How often?" and "How long?" to gauge your time commitment on a routine basis (daily or monthly).

Don't get caught off guard about the location of the trial or study site. Find out if you'll have to travel to another town, hospital, or state to participate. If you are the caregiver, it's important to factor in this additional logistical complications and time commitment to your existing time-management challenges.

7. What kind of support will I/we receive during the trial?

Find out in advance what your insurance carrier will cover if you participate in this clinical trial and what costs will come out of your own pocket. Don't forget incidental costs, like additional child care, time off from work, or transportation costs, which can add up over time. You want to be compensated for your time and inconvenience either by your insurance carrier or the study's sponsors. Trials often pay for the doctors' visits, medications, blood work, and diagnostics that are part of the study. Know exactly who pays what and if you are getting paid before you sign anything.

You also want to know the details of how the patient's health and well-being will be monitored during the trial. Find out if there's a system of safeguards in place for any problems that occur during the trial. Ask if you/your loved one will be allowed to move from the standard treatment group to the experimental one if the new drug is clearly superior.

Ask, "Who will be my medical team?" "Who can I call if I have questions?" "Who will be in charge of my care during the trial, especially if I experience side effects?" "Can I join support groups or talk about this trial if I want to?" "Will there be support for my family during the trial?" "How will my medical records and confidentiality be protected?" Also ask, "Who will cover the cost of any health care necessary if there are complications or serious side effects from the treatment?"

8. What will happen when the trial ends?

Be sure you understand what kind (if any) of follow-up medical support there is after the trial ends. Can you expect to receive medical care or some other kind of support follow-up care?

Ask, "Will I/we have any post-trial responsibilities?" and "Who will be responsible for the post-trial segment of this study?" Sometimes the new drug or treatment is so useful that participants want to continue with it even after the trial ends.

Find out if this will be an option for you. Ask, "Can I opt to remain on this treatment even after termination of the trial?" "Will I have to pay for medications to continue and if so, how much will it cost?" Lastly, you probably will want to know about how the study turned out. Find out how you will get the results at the trial's conclusion.

9. What happens if the person with AD is harmed by the trial? Can I/my loved one freely withdraw at any time without penalty?

Don't neglect to examine the worst-case scenario about patient safety. Ask, "What will happen if I have complications as the result of this study?" "Who will be responsible?" "How will the trial sponsors be held accountable?" and "Who will pay for my medical expenses if I'm injured?"

You also want to know the details about leaving the study early, either by your choice or if you are asked to leave. If you leave early, find out if you'll have to seek treatment elsewhere and if there will be any restrictions on your future treatments.

Researchers do everything in their power to make certain you complete the study, but there are a few circumstances where you might be asked to leave early. For example, there may be a change in your health status that makes it dangerous for you to participate, or you may be unable to follow the prescribed protocol. Ask about the conditions and provisions for withdrawal. Your informed consent form should spell out an escape clause.

Pathologist and Alzheimer's expert Dr. Roger A. Brumback says, "Humans aren't just big mice, so you must be cautious. Many trials results are overblown. There are legitimate studies, but they are just preliminary. Be very cautious about what's advertised."

Many times a researcher's salary is based on the number of patients he enrolls in a study. This can be a dangerous conflict of interest and result in enrolling people who might not be proper candidates or keep people in a study despite serious side effects.

10. Am I/my loved one a good candidate? Why or why not? What is your recommendation?

Ask your doctor to summarize your discussion with her about clinical trials by finding out if you or your loved one is a good candidate, both from a medical perspective and in terms of eligibility.

Stay alert to any possible bias on your doctor's part due to her own participation in a certain trial. You can phrase the question as something like, "If you weren't doing this research, what would

AM I/MY LOVED ONE RIGHT FOR A CLINICAL TRIAL?

Before volunteering for a clinical trial, you need to do your homework to assess your readiness and willingness to be an Alzheimer's guinea pig. These following questions work equally well for caregivers and for people with early stage AD.

1. **What are my personal goals for wanting to participate in a clinical trial?** Be honest with yourself about your own motivations.

2. **How far am I willing to go?** Answer this question based on your own tolerance for taking risks and how serious your diagnosis is.

3. **Do I have the time needed to participate in a clinical trial?** Some clinical trials are time consuming and may take years, while others are much shorter.

4. **How important is it to me that I work with my current doctor?** If your current doctor is not part of the clinical trial, you may need to find a new doctor who is.

5. **Am I confident and comfortable with the goals of this study and with the staff at the research center?** Ideally, the trial's goals match your personal values and the staff will treat you and your loved one well.

6. **How important is it to me to help other people with Alzheimer's disease?**
   Participating in a clinical trial is a way of helping future generations of AD patients if this is your thing.

7. **How will this trial affect my daily life?** Logistical concerns include travel time and expenses, child care needs, and time off from work.

8. **Will my family and loved one support my decision to participate in this clinical trial?** Talk over your interests and the clinical trial's requirements with the other people in your life who might be affected.

9. **Have I read the informed consent document and taken enough time to truly understand it?** Has everything been adequately explained to me? Be sure to ask about anything that's unclear to you, especially if you have MCI or early stage AD and find the fine print and technicalities to be confusing.

10. **How realistic am I about what I have to gain personally from participating?** Don't answer this question in a vacuum of knowledge about this trial you are considering.

you say is best for me?" If you feel pressured to participate, go get an objective second opinion from a doctor not connected to this doctor or with the trial. See chapter 5 on second opinions.

THE QUESTION DOCTOR SAYS:

Ask lots of questions before you sign anything, especially about the fine print in the informed consent document. If you are the person with AD, be patient with yourself until you understand this form entirely. And the same is true if you are the caregiver giving consent for your loved one. These documents can be confusing for even the most highly intelligent people.

❯ The Magic Question

Are there any other things I need to know about why the researchers are recruiting volunteers for this clinical trial? If you don't know, how can I find out more?

Doctors and research centers recommend specific clinical trials for a variety of reasons. While the vast majority of reasons involve purely humanitarian and scientific interests, there are a few rare exceptions. Some trials have trouble attracting enough participants and have to advertise to recruit volunteers.

Find out specifically why there haven't been enough volunteers before you commit to a trial. It could be that the trial simply requires a larger number of participants than the researchers or AD centers can recruit from their own patients, or there could be other factors like a long time commitment required from volunteers.

Think of this question as your "better safe than sorry" question before participating in a clinical trial.

CONCLUSION

Each person's experience in a clinical trial is unique. Two people with the same diagnosis and stage of Alzheimer's disease, receiving the same treatments in the same place and time, won't always react the same way to the treatment they receive during a clinical trial. Today's standard treatments were yesterday's clinical trials.

THE 10 BEST RESOURCES

Alzheimer's Association. "Clinical Studies." www.alz.org/alzheimers_disease_clinical_studies.asp.

Alzheimer's Association. "Clinical Trials Index." www.alz.org/alzheimers_disease_clinical_trials_index.asp.

Alzheimer's Disease Education and Referral Center. "Clinical Trials." www.nia.nih.gov/Alzheimers/ResearchInformation/ClinicalTrials. (Database of current trials.)

Centerwatch. Lists more than 41,000 trials mainly conducted by the pharmaceutical industry. Search by therapeutic category or condition. www.centerwatch.com

ClinicalTrials.gov. A comprehensive registry of federally and privately supported clinical trials in the United States and worldwide. www.clinicaltrials.gov.

ClinicalTrials.gov. "Understanding Clinical Trials." www.clinicaltrials.gov/ct2/info/understand.

ECRI. "Should I Enter a Clinical Trial? A Patient Reference Guide for Adults with a Serious or Life-Threatening Illness." www.ecri.org/Documents/Clinical_Trials_Patient_Reference_Guide.pdf.

Getz, Ken, and Deborah Borfitz. *Informed Consent: The Consumer's Guide to the Risks and Benefits of Volunteering for Clinical Trials.* Boston: CenterWatch, 2002.

National Institute on Aging. "Clinical Trials" (lists current trials). www
.nia.nih.gov/HealthInformation/ClinicalTrials.htm.

Wikipedia. "Clinical trial." http://en.wikipedia.org/wiki/clinical_trial.

PART III:

Caring for the Person with Alzheimer's Disease

The gradual, irreversible changes in the brain caused by Alzheimer's disease that affect a person's cognitive abilities also diminish the basic reasoning capabilities that most of us take for granted. This means that over time people with AD lose their ability to live alone and take care of themselves. Unfortunately, they may not fully realize the extent of their decline or they may be in denial about their worsening symptoms, confusion, and agitation.

The seven chapters in this section provide practical advice and support for caregivers at each step along the way. This section is arranged according to the person's increasing care needs. Chapter 10 helps you to determine if your loved one can remain living in his or her own home. Use chapter 11 to assess that home for safety. The goal of chapter 12 is to help you decide if you should care for your elderly parent in your own home.

Most caregivers finally realize they can't do it all and seek outside, part-time professional caregiving to supplement their own efforts. Choosing an adult day care center and/or a home health care agency is discussed in chapters 13 and 14 and represents this usual next step in caregiving. Ask these Best Questions to help guarantee that you hire the best services available in your area.

As your loved one's AD progresses beyond home care, chapter 15 presents the Best Questions to ask the directors of long-term care facilities, including nursing homes and assisted living residences, to make a wise and cost-effective decision. There is also a checklist of the Best Questions to ask yourself as you tour these facilities, which will alert you to the warning signs of potential problems you might otherwise overlook.

And lastly, chapter 16 lists the Best Questions to ask yourself as you assess whether or not your loved one in a long-term care residence has been—or could be—the victim of physical, emotional, or financial elder abuse. This is a serious worry for many families. These questions may ease your concerns or alert you to the need to investigate further.

As you journey from your loved one's living independently to dependency in a long-term care environment, each set of 10 Best Questions in this section will help you to cut through the complexities and empower you to make the best care decisions possible.

CHAPTER 10

THE 10 BEST QUESTIONS

to Decide if Your Loved One Can
Remain at Home

> In the end, it's not the years in your life that count. It's the
> life in your years.
>
> —Abraham Lincoln

I f you are like most caregivers, you agonize over whether or not
your loved one can remain living at home. This is true whether
or not you live with your loved one—either as a spouse or as an
adult child who has brought your parent into your own home—
or if you are a long-distance caregiver worrying about your parent
living alone in another state. A burning question for many caregivers is, "How much longer can my loved one stay at home?"

According to the Family Caregiver Alliance, there are more
than 52 million informal and family caregivers in the United States.
The Alzheimer's Association states that there were nearly 10 million adult Americans providing 8.4 billion hours of unpaid care to
people with Alzheimer's disease in 2007. Unpaid family caregiving
continues to be the largest source of long-term care services in the
United States and is expected to increase by 85 percent between
2000 and 2050 as the baby boom generation ages.

Most people with early to middle-stage Alzheimer's disease depend on their family and friends to get through the day. The vast
majority of U.S. adults (78 percent) in long-term care receive all
their care from unpaid family and friends. An estimated 59 to 75
percent of caregivers are female, mostly wives and adult daughters.
Another 14 percent of caregiving is a combination of family care
and paid help, such as home health care aides, part-time skilled
nurses, or adult day care services.

With cost of a private room in a nursing home soaring to above $74,000 a year, as cited in MetLife's 2005 national nursing home study and rising by at least 6 percent each year, according to a New York Life Insurance study, along with the negative stigma most associate with nursing home care, families want to keep their loved one at home as long as possible. In addition, the person with mild to moderate AD is usually more comfortable on familiar turf and is less likely to become agitated or confused if they can remain at home.

This chapter's list of 10 Best Questions is designed to help you make a well-educated decision about keeping your loved one at home. But remember, it's important that you speak to your doctor before you make any final decisions.

There are also specially trained professionals—such as geriatric care managers, certified aging-in-place specialists, nurses, and occupational therapists—who can help you make a more definitive analysis of your loved one's ability to remain at home. The Best Questions in this chapter are not meant to be a substitute for these professionals' evaluations and advice.

Personal safety is the first and foremost consideration when you are deciding if your loved one can remain at home. Because of its importance, safety is considered in depth separately in chapter 11.

The Best Questions in this chapter are based on the standardized assessment criteria used by medical professionals, called the **Activities of Daily Living (ADLs).** Activities of Daily Living are basic self-care tasks, like one's ability to eat, bathe, and dress. ADLs are judged on a continuum assessment scale that ranges from "fully independent/needs no assistance" to "needs some assistance" to "unable to do without help from others." There are other important tasks, called **Instrumental Activities of Daily Living (IADLs),** such as preparing meals, shopping, or managing money, that are less crucial because they can be delegated to others. Health professionals, nursing homes, and health insurance providers routinely use ADLs and IADLs to measure a person's functional status and independence.

Consider your loved one's living arrangements. Is he living alone or with others? A person with AD who lives alone with few outside resources for help will need higher-level ADL capabilities in order to remain at home than someone who has a full-time caregiver living in the same home with him.

The first four Best Questions are based on ADLs and are the most crucial to assess a person's capacity for independent living. The last six Best Questions and the Magic Question are based on IADLs. Their importance varies depending on whether or not zthe person with AD lives alone and has a part-time or full-time caregiver or paid assistance. Each Best Question has three bullets which list the capabilities that correspond to this simplified functional assessment scale:

- Needs no assistance
- Needs some assistance
- Unable to do

THE QUESTION DOCTOR SAYS:

Since people with AD often have good days and bad days, as you are working through this assessment, you may want to evaluate your loved one every day over a week or ten days for each Best Question, rather than just perform a one-time assessment. This will give you a clearer picture of your loved one's true functional capabilities and ability to remain at home.

>>> THE 10 BEST QUESTIONS
to Decide if Your Loved One Can Remain at Home

1. How well can my loved one handle his own personal hygiene, bathing, and dressing?

The ability to dress and groom oneself independently is a prime factor when considering keeping your loved one in his home. If the person with AD has a full-time caregiver who lives in the same home, independence in hygiene, bathing, and dressing is of less concern than for people with AD who are living alone or have only part-time assistance.

Ask yourself if your loved one:

- Routinely performs all daily bathing, dressing, and shaving activities without assistance? (Needs no/some assistance)
- Requires reminders about daily hygiene, help with shoe-laces, zippers, hooks, etc.? (Needs no/some assistance)
- Depends on others for most or all personal hygiene, bathing, and dressing activities? (Unable to do)

2. How capable is my loved one of eating, choosing nutritious food, and preparing meals independently?

The ability to eat without assistance is a key activity of daily life. If your loved one is living alone or has only part-time caregiving, she needs a higher degree of independence than someone who can depend on others for eating assistance or meal preparation.

The ability to prepare nutritious meals for oneself is also important, but to a lesser extent when community support services are available. These include Meals on Wheels (www.mowaa.org), a senior nutrition program operating in the United States, Canada, and Australia, or the UK-based National Association of Care Catering (www.thenacc.co.uk). Check out Volunteers of America (www.volunteersofamerica.org) or local services available through your church or synagogue.

For AD caregivers, mealtimes can be a challenging battle-ground. Your loved one may have a poor appetite, forget to eat, or forget that she has already eaten. Try to establish and stick with regular mealtimes, limit distractions, check the food's temperature, and serve simple foods one at a time.

Consider whether the person with AD can shop independently or needs to be accompanied on routine grocery errands. Some people lose their understanding of money, while others may be too frail to carry packages. In some regions there are shopping services or stores that will deliver groceries to your home.

Does my loved one:

- Plan, prepare, and eat adequately nutritious meals without assistance?
- Rely on meals prepared by others or require assistance when eating (opening containers, pouring, cutting, etc.)?
- Need total assistance from others for nourishment or re-minders to eat?

3. How independent is my loved one with his toilet needs and continence?

The National Association for Continence defines incontinence as the involuntary loss of bladder or bowel control. This is a common problem among Alzheimer's patients with progressed-disease symptoms and a key decision criterion for many caregivers about whether or not they can continue to care for their loved one at home. A person's degree of incontinence can also determine eligibility for adult day care centers, professional in-home care arrangements, or assisted living facilities.

Does my loved one:

- Demonstrate complete and independent continence on a daily basis?
- Have occasional incontinence, a colostomy, or catheter, but can still manage with self-toileting or require only occasional assistance?
- Have daily, uncontrollable incontinence and lack the ability to communicate about it?

4. How mobile is my loved one around the house?

In the language of a formal ADL functional assessment, mobility is often called *transferring*. Transferring means the person's ability to move around inside the home, including such basic tasks as moving unassisted from the bed to a chair or to use the bathroom.

Consider if your loved one needs (or will soon need) a wheelchair, cane, or walker. Your home's long stairways or narrow doorways may not be well suited or easy to retrofit to accommodate someone who is physically disabled.

Does my loved one:

- Move independently from a chair, toilet, or bed?
- Rely on a cane, walker, or wheelchair or require some assistance due to occasional confusion or physical disability?
- Require full transfer assistance, including turning in bed and moving to and from a wheelchair?

5. Can my loved one do housekeeping and personal laundry chores?

Some experts believe this is an optional IADL for a person who has a full-time caregiver or can afford to pay someone else to perform cleaning and laundry tasks. Historically, this IADL was excluded for men.

However, if your loved one lives alone—and especially if she lives in an older house that needs regular maintenance and upkeep—this can be a major concern. For example, you may be a long-distance caregiver who worries constantly about your parents' home falling into a state of disrepair beyond routine care.

Does my loved one:

- Maintain the house alone to an acceptable level of cleanliness and repair with occasional outside help for gardening, painting, etc.?
- Do light daily/weekly tasks such as dishwashing, most personal laundry, straightening, and bed making at an acceptable level of cleanliness but not do heavy cleaning or maintenance?
- Need all home maintenance tasks, light housekeeping, and personal laundry to be done by others?

6. Can my loved one be fully trusted to always take her medications as prescribed?

It's important that your loved one can remember to take any drugs for Alzheimer's disease as well as medications for other conditions, such as heart disease, diabetes, or glaucoma. For many elderly people, their daily regime involves a complex dispensing schedule and a full handful of pills.

Even well-intended people with AD who are starting to slip mentally can't remember if they have already taken today's pills or not. As the caregiver, you need to ensure your loved one is getting proper medications and won't be harmed by incorrect dosing. People with AD and living alone are at high risk for medication problems.

Does my loved one:

- Take her correct medications in the correct dosages at the correct times every day?

- Show responsibility for self-medication if the drugs are pre-packed or prepared in advance in separate dosages or make only minor or occasional dosing errors?
- Become routinely confused or prove to be incapable of self-medication?

7. How well can my loved one handle personal finances?

If your loved one lives alone, pays others for in-home care services, or still maintains the household budget and bill-paying duties, it's imperative that he be able to manage money well and without mental impairment. The gradual loss of "money smarts" is what often leads to the headline-grabbing stories of elderly people having their lifetime savings stolen by a con artist or through a telephone, television, or Internet scam.

Evelyn, a full-time caregiver in Little Rock, Arkansas, reflects on her experiences during the last three years caring for her middle-stage AD husband, Robert. "I've tried to walk a fine line between giving him as much independence as I could but have always been on the lookout, too. Robert thinks he's fine, but often he's not. It's just hard for him to realize he can't do these things anymore."

When the person with AD has a full-time caregiver who is totally responsible for the household money management, then this IADL becomes less important.

Does my loved one:

- Manage financial matters independently (can write checks, pay bills, go to the bank, and balance the checkbook)?
- Keep track of day-to-day purchases but need some help with banking and major purchases?
- Become totally confused about finances and is incapable of handling money?

8. How capable is my loved one of using some form of transportation for short trips, to go shopping, or to run errands?

This measure of independence is called **mode of transportation.** People with early stage AD may still be able to get around fairly well, including driving. Once someone with AD can no longer drive, public transportation may be a viable option, depending on where he lives and his past familiarity with the bus, train, or taxi system.

If your loved one travels around town, you may find some peace of mind if he is wearing a medical alert identification. There are also local and national transportation services for the elderly that can suggest alternative methods of transportation. Check with your local Alzheimer's Association or Beverly Foundation (www.beverly foundation.org) for community-based transportation services. See chapter 22 for more on transportation.

Does my loved one:

- Travel independently on public transportation or safely drive his own car?
- No longer drive but can arrange his own travel via public transportation or taxi?
- Have little or no ability to travel without assistance from others due to mental confusion or physical problems?

9. How mentally aware was my loved in the last few weeks?

This Best Question is a general-assessment question for live-at-home caregivers or for long-distance caregivers who have recently talked with their loved one by telephone.

If you are a long-distance caregiver, reflect on how well your loved one uses the telephone as an indicator of mental alertness. If your loved one can operate the phone, including looking up phone numbers and dialing, this is a positive sign of alertness compared to someone who answers the phone, but can't dial it or becomes totally confused while on the phone. See more Best Questions for long-distance caregivers in chapter 19.

Does my loved one:

- Show the ability to reason and remember with only occasional memory lapses?
- Require some assistance during increasing periods of confusion, disorientation, or poor judgment?
- Demonstrate severely impaired orientation, memory, and judgment skills or is unable to follow directions?

10. How well could my loved one respond to an emergency that required quick action or evacuation of the home?

Many caregivers focus on just getting through another day without thinking about worst-case scenarios, like a home fire or explosion or natural disaster such as floods, tornadoes, hurricanes, or severe snowstorms. Just consider the aftermath of Hurricane Katrina on the unprepared elderly people living in New Orleans who were caught in this deadly disaster.

If your loved one is not fully mobile, uses a wheelchair or walker, or is especially frail or heavyset, you need to think in advance about whether you have the physical strength to carry him out of your home in case of emergency. This is especially critical if you live in a region that is prone to seasons of hurricanes, floods, or tornadoes. If your loved one lives alone or you are a long-distance caregiver, ask yourself, What would happen to her in an emergency? Who could help her?

Does my loved one:

- Understand and is capable of the proper evacuation procedures in case of emergency?
- Rely on a cane, walker, or wheelchair and would need assistance during an emergency?
- Have such severely impaired judgment that he would be totally dependent during an emergency?

❯ The Magic Question

How long can I, as the caregiver, continue to support my loved one at home without it endangering my own health and well-being?

If your live-in loved one is in the bottom assessment category for some or most of the above Best Questions, especially questions 1 through 4, you need to take a long, hard look at the realities of finding alternative care for her while also taking good care of yourself, too.

To keep your loved one at home, a lot depends on your personal time, your own mental and physical health, and your reservoir of energy for this very demanding job of full-time caregiving.

Clare Absher, an experienced geriatric nurse and consultant in Kitty Hawk, North Carolina, comments, "Caring for your loved one with Alzheimer's at home initially is often the best option. It is less traumatic because the loved one is in familiar surroundings. The key factor is that there has to be a willing and able caregiver, one solid family member or friend."

CONCLUSION

The decision to keep your loved one at home isn't a one-time event. It's an assumption that will be continually challenged by her changing needs, new circumstances, and the mental and physical decline caused by the progression of Alzheimer's disease. Sometimes you'll know what to do without having a professional assessment, as caregiver Elaine Marshall of Leesburg, Virginia, recalls before her mother with Alzheimer's moved in with Elaine's family. "It's so hard when the person is still pretty much aware and thinks they can be on their own. But you *know* they can't be and to allow it would be negligent."

You don't have to make this decision alone. Ask your doctor and seek other specialized assistance. Using part-time paid home health care nurses or aides and adult day care services will also help you keep your loved one at home longer because these professionals can relieve you from constant caregiving chores.

In the movie classic *The Wizard of Oz,* Dorothy said it best when she told her little dog, Toto, "There's no place like home." Yes, Dorothy, that's so true—but then again, Toto didn't have Alzheimer's disease.

THE 10 BEST RESOURCES

AARP. "Certified Aging-in-Place Specialists." www.aarp.org/families/home_design/rate_home/a2004-03-23-caps.html.

Alternatives for Seniors. "Evaluation Tool." www.alternativesforseniors.com/Evaluation.aspx.

Brawley, Elizabeth C. *Design Innovations for Aging and Alzheimer's.* New York: John Wiley & Sons, 2005.

Laurenhue, Kathy. *Activities of Daily Living: An ADL Guide for Alzheimer's Care.* Bradenton, Fla.: Wiser Now, 2006.

Mace, Nancy, and Peter Rabins. "Problems in Independent Living." In *The 36-Hour Day: A Family Guide to Caring for Persons with Alzheimer's Disease, Related Dementing Illnesses, and Memory Loss in Later Life,* 4th ed. Baltimore, Md.: The Johns Hopkins University Press, 2006.

MetLife. "Family Caregiving." www.metlife.com/FileAssets/MMI/MMISYC FamilyCaregiving2007.pdf.

National Association of Home Builders. "Hire a Certified Aging-in-Place Specialist (CAPS)." www.nahb.org/generic.aspx?sectionID=717&generic ContentID=8484.

U.S. Department of Health and Human Services, Administration on Aging. "Emergency Readiness for Older Adults and Caregivers." www.aoa .gov/PROF/aoaprog/caregiver/overview/Just_in_Case030706_links.pdf.

U.S. Department of Homeland Security, FEMA, and American Red Cross. "Preparing for Disaster for People with Disabilities and Other Special Needs." www.redcross.org/images/pdfs/preparedness/A4497.pdf.

Wallace, Meredith, and Mary Shelkey. "Katz Index of Independence in Activities of Daily Living (ADL)." *Try This,* Issue 2, revised 2007. www .hartfordign.org/publications/trythis/issue02.pdf.

CHAPTER 11: THE 10 BEST QUESTIONS

to Assess Home Safety for a Loved One with Alzheimer's Disease

> Step with care and great tact
> And remember that Life's a Great Balancing Act
> Just never forget to be dexterous and deft
> And never mix up your right foot with your left.
>
> —Dr. Seuss, *Oh, the Places You'll Go*

The most desirable situation for most Alzheimer's patients and their families is loving care at home. But this is impossible without home safety. Making sure that your loved one's home is safe and injury proof is crucial, especially since most AD patients are also elderly and suffer from losses in vision, hearing, mobility, and strength.

For your loved one to remain at home for as long as possible, it's imperative that you have a home safety assessment. This assessment is best done by professionals, such as occupational therapists, physical therapists, or geriatric care managers, who will visit your home, identify safety hazards, and suggest improvements and modifications. Contact your local Alzheimer's Association office for referrals.

The following 10 Best Questions will give you a quick overview of potential home safety hazards and have been derived from dozens of safety checklists tailored for seniors and other sources cited in the Resources section (page 273). Rate each safety consideration in your loved one's home on this three-point scale:

1. Adequate, needs few or no changes
2. Needs minor or low-cost changes

3. Represents a major safety hazard that needs immediate attention

Simple and cost-effective solutions are included for making the home safer and more accessible for a person with Alzheimer's disease.

These Best Questions should not be used as a substitute for a professional home safety evaluation. Richard of Las Vegas, Nevada, remembers, "It was a struggle to get my dad to understand that it was not safe for him at home anymore and get him evaluated. He realized it might mean the end to his independence."

❯❯❯ THE 10 BEST QUESTIONS
to Assess Home Safety for a Loved One with Alzheimer's Disease

1. How safe and accessible are the exterior steps, doors, and walkways? What can I do to make the home exterior safer for my loved one?

To improve access in and out of the home, install permanent or temporary ramps, widen doorways to accompany a wheelchair or walker, and install swing-clear hinges on the doors. Exterior steps are a major source of life-threatening falls for the elderly or confused, so make sure they are sturdy and in good repair. Install sturdy guardrails and handrails on all exterior steps. Ensure that the steps, entry landings, porches, and decks are all well lit and easily accessible.

Look carefully at the walkways leading up to the home. Are they clear and free of slippery grass or overhanging shrubs; the surfaces smooth, even, and not too steep; and the walkway length and width easy for someone with a walking impairment or wheelchair? Is the pathway to the car in the driveway or garage clutter free and clearly marked?

If you spot potential problems, ask a professional landscaper, design expert, or handyman for help in making improvements.

2. How safe and accessible are the interior steps, doors, and hallways? What can I do to make these areas safer?

You can make the interior stairs easier and safer for your loved one by installing handrails, using nonskid, reflective rubber strips and glow tape, ensuring the steps are well lit, not too steep or shallow, and that their edges are clearly visible. Replace doorknobs with lever handles, check that the thresholds are low and smooth and that doorways can accommodate a wheelchair, if necessary.

The interior hallways need light switches at both ends and should be free of obstacles. Consider widening hallways or installing handrails for unsteady loved ones.

3. Where are the areas in the home (inside and out) most likely to cause my loved one to fall? What can I do to prevent my loved one from falling?

For the elderly, a fall can be a life-altering event. Falls may lead to serious fractures, permanent disabilities, or death. According to MetLife, every year more than one-third of older people fall, and up to 30 percent of those falls result in moderate to severe injuries. Falls are the leading cause of injuries seen in hospital emergency rooms and the most common accident occurring at home. AARP found that 78 percent of elderly falls occur inside or near the home. Older adults who have fallen are four to five times more likely to be admitted to a nursing home afterward.

Rearrange furniture to keep pathways clear. All doormats, carpet runners, and pads should be tacked down or have nonskid backing and no upturned corners. Tile and bare wooden floors should be slip resistant, especially for old feet in socks. Other safety features include secured railings, well-lit rooms and exterior areas, nightlights, and grab bars and shower seats for the bathroom. Get your loved one a cane, walker, and rubber-soled shoes to help steady his gait.

Each room should have a clear, unobstructed pathway without clutter, cords, wires, baskets, or other things to trip over. Pay close attention to the flooring. The proper flooring can reduce the risk of falls, promote mobility and comfort, and enhance safety.

Design experts favor installed carpeting, which provides a smooth surface, prevents slippage, reduces irritating noise levels and glare, and cushions any falls that do occur. Flooring with large, contrasting patterns, like a rug with giant diamonds or flowers, can be disorienting and impair balance.

4. Where are potential fire hazards in the home? What can I do to minimize the possibility of my loved one starting a fire?

The Home Safety Council reports that fires and burns are the third leading cause of unintentional home injuries. When someone with AD lives in the home, the risk of fire can skyrocket if safety measures are not installed. You may need to use locked covers on the stove burners, put matches behind childproof locks, or keep the kitchen off-limits entirely.

Invest in a good-quality fire extinguisher. Smoke detectors and carbon monoxide alarms should be properly installed and checked monthly to ensure they are in good working order. Create an exit plan for the home with a simple diagram for your loved one. Practice your escape plan with your loved one at least twice, once during the day and again at night.

5. What is potentially unsafe in the bathroom? What can I do to correct any safety problems there?

Many older people are at risk each time they use their home bathrooms. Modifications for support in the bathroom can be as simple as installing sturdy grab bars in the shower and around the toilet (don't use regular towel bars), installing shower seats or transfer benches, using a hand-held shower head and a raised toilet seat, gluing nonskid strips to the floor of the shower or tub, and substituting dual-control (hot-cold) for single-control faucets. Install an antiscald device on the hot water heater or turn it down.

Consider replacing glass shower enclosures with nonbreakable materials. Make sure the room is free of tripping hazards, like an overly long shower curtain, general clutter, or small scatter rugs. Ensure that the room is properly heated and cooled (AD patients are often sensitive to temperature extremes) and that the floor is not slippery when wet. All medicines, razors, and other harmful objects should be hidden away or secured in cabinets with child-proof locks.

Check that the toilet seat is securely fastened. You may also want to use bath fixtures of contrasting colors or post instructions by the shower, sink, or toilet to help if your loved one becomes easily confused.

6. What are potential safety problems in the bedroom? What can I do to improve these problems?

Your loved one may benefit from having a photo or memento on the bedroom door to help recognize her own bedroom. The bed should be at proper height with easy access and a night light nearby. A clear, well-lit path to the toilet is needed that is free of cords, wires, or other hazards. Ideally, the bedroom will have at least one comfortable chair that is safe and easy to get in and out of for elderly people. Windows should be fire-escape accessible and easy to open (or securely locked if wandering is a problem).

Tables need to have rounded edges. Avoid furniture with rolling wheels. Remove colognes, after-shave lotions, and other potentially dangerous items from dresser tops. Blinds, shades, and curtains should operate easily, be securely attached, and be short enough avoid tripping problems. Closets and drawers should be easy to open and sliding glass doors secured on their tracks.

Consider labeling drawers and closets to help your loved one find personal items more easily. Some caregivers use baby monitors or intercoms for extra peace of mind at night.

7. How well is the home lit inside and out? What can be done about the home's lighting that will improve my loved one's ability to see well?

Check for adequate lighting in the driveway, garage, walkways, at all doors, and throughout all most-frequented living areas. Each room needs an accessible light switch by the door.

Many caregivers don't realize how much glare and reflection can contribute to confusion, agitation, or anger. For example, glare on a wooden floor can cause an older person with impaired vision or judgment to fear falling. Older eyes don't adjust as well to intense lights or brightness, so make the appropriate changes around the home, from overhead lights to table lamps. Multidirectional lighting creates more even illumination. Place night lights in the hallways and other high-traffic areas.

8. Are all potentially dangerous items in the kitchen safely secured?

The kitchen holds a vast potential for harm, including poisons, hot pans, boiling water, fire, sharp objects, and an unlocked refrigerator or freezer. According to the American Association of Poison Control Centers, accidental poisoning is the second leading cause of home-related, unintentional deaths. Use childproof locks on the drawers or cabinets to protect your loved one from sharp knives, poisonous substances like household cleaners and bleach, electric appliances such as a blender, mixer, or an electric knife, and all vitamins, prescription drugs, and over-the-counter medicines.

Be sure to control access to the stove and microwave oven by removing the knobs, locking the oven door, or installing a hidden circuit breaker or gas valve. Remove any items that resemble food, like wax fruit, food-shaped magnets, or other countertop knick-knacks. Keep the kitchen free of clutter both at countertop and floor levels.

Clearly and simply label the drawers and cabinets that hold allowable items. If your loved one has advanced Alzheimer's, consider closing off access to the kitchen entirely because of the potential hazards for fire, burns, cuts, and poisoning.

9. Does my loved one have a history of wandering away from home? If so, what can I do to prevent it in the future?

Wandering is one of the most frightening symptoms of advanced Alzheimer's disease. It only takes a moment for your loved one to wander away. The Alzheimer's Association estimates that nearly 60 percent of AD patients wander. Many people with AD can't remember their names, home addresses, familiar places and faces, or how to get back home.

Ideally, look for a safe outdoor place that your loved one can use without wandering, such as an escape-proof porch or fenced-in yard with a locked gate. AD experts now believe that many wanderers are actually trying to go someplace in their own minds.

Install security locks on all exterior doors (requiring a double key or with the lock installed out of sight), use childproof doorknobs, camouflage doors, and hide a key outside in case the caregiver gets locked out by the person with AD. Control off-limits areas like storage sheds or basements with locks or security gates. Make sure all windows are securely locked.

You may want to install motion sensors or alarms on exterior doors or in the yard. Make sure that there are eye-level decals or other warning signs on all large picture windows and sliding glass doors so your loved one doesn't accidentally walk into the glass.

10. Would my loved one be safer if she had a medical alert device?

There are hundreds of providers of medical alert devices, identification bracelets and necklaces, and telephone and emergency response systems. A simple and often low-cost device or arrangement might be an added safety advantage for your loved one while giving you valuable peace of mind, especially if she is a wanderer. Ask your doctor or local Alzheimer's support group for recommendations.

The Alzheimer's Association offers a program called MedicAlert + Safe Return, which features a twenty-four-hour nationwide emergency response service for individuals with AD who wander off or have a medical emergency.

❯ The Magic Question

What have I forgotten to secure in my loved one's home if he were a child?

Imagine that you are trying to protect a young child from harm in the home. A person with AD often becomes childlike as her ability to understand what's safe and what isn't erodes away with the disease's progression.

If your loved one lives with you, this question might be even tougher to answer. The very thing that could be the biggest safety hazard might be in clear sight, right under your nose, or tucked away and long forgotten. If you have lived in your home a long time, you may not have thought about what changes are needed. Now you need to reconsider your home as if you had children (again).

Candidates for this category include guns or other weapons,

plastic or dry cleaning bags that could cause suffocation, alcohol, and poisonous plants (check with your local gardening or extension service). Install childproof plugs on all unused electrical outlets. Cover any overly hot or cold surfaces such as radiators, hot water pipes, and air conditioning units. Make sure your loved one can use the telephone, or consider buying him an emergency alert device instead.

If you have a swimming pool, ensure that access to it is restricted. Secure your lawnmower, other electrical gardening equipment, outdoor grills, home computers, and any valuable disks, papers, or computer equipment. Install gates across the doorways to rooms where you want to limit access. Make sure there is a well-stocked first aid kit on hand but off-limits to the person with AD.

If there are pets in the home, protect their safety as well. Make sure pets can't be harmed by your loved one. For example, caged birds, fish, or small dogs or cats might become unintentional victims without your intervention, forethought, and preventive measures.

THE QUESTION DOCTOR SAYS:

Don't make your home safety assessment a one-time event. A quick review of these Best Questions weekly or monthly, especially for falls and fire hazards, may be a lifesaver.

CONCLUSION

As a caregiver, two of your most important responsibilities are to identify safety hazards in the home and to recognize the point when your loved one is no longer safe living there. As author Jacqueline Marcell says, "You have to put your loved one's safety first. No matter how much he protests. Don't wait for a heartbreaking accident and the overwhelming guilt for not taking charge when you knew what needed to be done."

Experienced geriatric nurse Clare Absher comments, "The deal breakers for keeping a loved one at home are to ask yourself, 'Can she recognize a dangerous situation? Can she use the telephone to call for help?' And 'Is she wandering?' "

Until you carefully look around or get a professional safety assessment, the home may be full of accidents just waiting to happen. By taking simple, low-cost actions, you can Alzheimer-proof the home and increase the time your loved one can remain there in safety and comfort. Getting a professional safety assessment along with using these 10 Best Questions will help you do the best job possible of making your loved one's home safe.

THE 10 BEST RESOURCES

Alzheimer's Association. "MedicAlert + Safe Return." Twenty-four-hour emergency response service. www.alz.org/we_can_help_medicalert_safe return.asp or call 1-888-572-8566.

Alzheimer's Association. "Wandering Behavior: Preparing for and Preventing It." www.alz.org/national/documents/topicsheet_wandering.pdf.

Alzheimer's Disease Education and Referral Service. "Home Safety for People with Alzheimer's Disease." www.nia.nih.gov/Alzheimers/Publica tions/homesafety.htm.

American Occupational Therapy Association. "Modifying Your Home for Independence." www.aota.org/Consumers/Tips/Adults/HomeMods/ 35132.aspx.

Brawley, Elizabeth C. *Designing for Alzheimer's Disease: Strategies for Creating Better Care Environments.* New York: John Wiley and Sons, 1997.

FamilyCare America. "Home Modification Checklist." www.caregivers library.org/Portals/0/HomeModificationChecklist.pdf.

Home Safety Council. "Think Safe Be Safe: Fire Prevention Tips." www
.homesafetycouncil.org/safety_guide/sg_fire_w001.aspx.

National Center for Injury Prevention and Control. "Home Safety Check-lists." www.cdc.gov/ncipc/falls/FallPrev4.pdf.

Senior Solutions of America. "Checklist: Is Your Loved One's Home Safe?"
www.aging-parents-and-elder-care.com/Pages/Checklists/Home_Safety_
Chklst.html.

Warner, Mark, and Ellen Warner. *The Complete Guide to Alzheimer's-Proofing Your Home.* West Lafayette, Ind.: Purdue University Press, 2000.

CHAPTER 12: THE 10 BEST QUESTIONS
to Decide, Should Mom Move In with Me?

What a drag it is getting old.

—Mick Jagger (in 1966 at age twenty-three)

L ike millions of other adult children with aging parents, you may harbor the idea that someday your mom or dad can "just come live with me." You've got a spare bedroom and it seems like an easy solution—until that "someday" becomes today and the reality of Alzheimer's disease sets in.

If your parent has a new diagnosis of early stage Alzheimer's disease or MCI, or if it's already too late for your father to live alone safely, you now face this decision; "Should my aging parent with Alzheimer's disease move in with me and my family?"

According to the Family Caregiver Alliance, about 25 percent of AD patients live with their adult children. Most caregivers (60 percent) have employment outside the home, including the baby boomers, who typically work and have younger family members to care for. Bringing your mom into your home is a big undertaking and responsibility, but it may seem like the only solution when you consider the costs of paid caregivers.

Perhaps so, but before you make a formal commitment, ask yourself the following Best Questions. These questions will help you to tackle this tough decision head-on. Try to be brutally honest in your answers and to look at all angles. Your emotions may be running high because you're worried about your mom's deteriorating condition, but try to make a rational decision that includes time for your reflections on how this may change your life.

> **THE QUESTION DOCTOR SAYS:**
>
> You may want to discuss these Best Questions with your immediate family, parents, other family members, or close friends to get their opinions, too. If you prefer, come up with your own Best Questions that need answers based on your family's situation.
>
> Then have a family meeting structured around Best Questions. Answering these questions will help you to stay focused and avoid conflicts. Invite a counselor or trusted friend to mediate if necessary.

>>> THE 10 BEST QUESTIONS
to Decide, Should Mom Move In with Me?

1. How much responsibility for my parent's care am I/we willing or capable of assuming?

Your answer has many variables, including your personal preferences, resources, and your mom's needs. This is a particularly hard question if you feel torn between your own family's needs and those of your increasingly fragile parent. Take into consideration your financial and emotional resources as well.

As Mayo Clinic's Alzheimer's expert Dr. Neill Graff-Radford says, "I think it's really important for the caregiver to look after her own health, for both the patient and the caregiver's sake. She shouldn't feel bad about wanting to look after her own health. It's not selfish, but actually a generous thing to do so she can help."

2. What does Mom want to do?

This answer depends on your mom's AD stage, her current living situation, how close your home is to hers, and her other housing options. There's no reason why you can't directly ask her this question

changes. Even if she's ambulatory, AD patients need special safety precautions in place to prevent them from wandering, hurting themselves, or setting the kitchen on fire. Even simple home renovations can be costly.

Use chapter 11 to evaluate home safety issues and adapt your home.

7. What outside support is available to help me care for Mom?

Check out your community's services for seniors, including adult day care, home health care services, and respite care. See chapters 13 and 14 for guidance. For example, knowing that you can take your mom to adult day care may mean you can keep your job.

Also explore family support and support groups (chapter 20). Lastly, look into the long-term care, assisted living, and nursing homes (chapter 15) in your area so you'll be more knowledgeable about these housing options as alternatives either now or later.

8. How much time do I/we have to make this decision?

If your mom has just been diagnosed with barely noticeable MCI, you have a less urgent decision than an adult child whose mom with moderate-stage Alzheimer's lives alone and has already burned herself. Try to rationally assess how long your mother can continue as she is. Hire an occupational therapist to help and see chapter 10 for guidance.

Your home circumstances may change, such as a grown child moving out, if you can afford to wait to have your mother move in. Just make sure your delay is not a denial of the situation and that your mom is safe for now.

9. What unresolved conflicts are there between me and my mom?

Most families have old hurts. For example, you may never have quite forgiven your mother for what she once said about your parenting skills or the man you married.

If you moved out of your mother's house twenty to forty years ago, you may have forgotten how rigid she can be or about her little annoying habits. Food preferences, personal habits like smoking or cleanliness, choice of friends, and religious beliefs are all potential areas of incompatibility and constant friction.

10. What will my/our day-to-day lives be like with Mom living here?

Try to imagine a routine day with her in your home. Mentally walk through the day from the point the morning alarm clock goes off to bedtime. How often did you interact with her? How did she change your normal routines? What happened for other family members living at home?

Once your mother's condition worsens, your daily life will be further complicated by constant caregiving chores. Many adult children feel awkward with this role reversal, especially giving physical care. Spoon-feeding Mom or washing Dad in the shower is not something you probably ever envisioned until now.

❯ The Magic Question

What will happen if Mom moves in, but it doesn't work out?

You need to consider this worst-case scenario now so you won't be caught totally by surprise if things don't turn out like you think they will.

Even some of the best intentions can sometimes go sour. You may be overwhelmed by your mom's worsening Alzheimer's behavioral symptoms, such as aggressiveness, wandering, and incontinence. She may refuse to eat or scream in the shower. Your husband or children at home may grow resentful of her disruptive presence in their lives. You may personally face financial hardships or depression. Managing a person with severe AD is a tremendous challenge even for the most capable caregiver.

Try to have a fallback plan. Research long-term care facilities at the same time you make the decision about your mom moving in. Talk to other family members about sharing the burden with you. Being realistic and organized in your decision making will help everyone.

CONCLUSION

The decision to invite your mom or father with Alzheimer's to move in with you should not be made hastily. If living in her own home isn't working out for your parent, it's important to consider all of the other options available, including your mother living with other siblings or relatives and long-term care. Having your mom or dad live with you can be an incredibly rewarding— and frustrating—experience.

Regardless of what ultimately happens, try to include everyone in this decision-making process, including your parents, spouse, siblings, and even young children to help ease any resentments or difficulties.

Invite your mother into your home because you want to and not from a sense of obligation only. Otherwise, you may be setting yourself up for a future of caregiver stress, depression, and burnout.

THE 10 BEST RESOURCES

Alzheimer's Association. "CareFinder." www.alz.org/carefinder/index.asp.

Alzheimer's Association. "Caregiving 101." www.alz.org/we_can_help_care giving101.asp.

Alzheimer's Association. "Caregiver Resources: Best Web Sites for Family Caregivers." www.alz.org/national/documents/Lib_Best_FCare.pdf.

Alzheimer's Disease Education and Referral Center. "Caregiver Guide." www.nia.nih.gov/Alzheimers/Publications/caregiverguide.htm.

Federal Citizen Information Center. "Life Advice About Caring for an Aging Loved One." www.pueblo.gsa.gov/cic_text/family/aging/loved ones.htm.

Henry, Stella, and Ann Convery. *The Eldercare Handbook: Difficult Choices, Compassionate Solutions.* New York: HarperCollins, 2006.

Loverde, Joy. "Caregivers." In *The Complete Eldercare Planner: Where to Start, Which Questions to Ask, and How to Find Help,* 2nd ed. New York: Three Rivers Press, 2000.

Mayo Clinic. "Alzheimer's: Dealing with Family Conflict." www.mayo clinic.com/health/alzheimers/AZ00027.

MetLife. "Alzheimer's Disease: Caregiving Challenges." www.metlife.com/ FileAssets/MMI/MMISYCAlzheimerCareChallenges07.pdf.

Morris, Virginia, and Robert M. Butler. *How to Care for Aging Parents.* New York: Workman Publishing, 2004.

CHAPTER 13: THE 10 BEST QUESTIONS
to Find Quality Adult Day Care
for Alzheimer's Patients

It takes a long time to grow young.

—Pablo Picasso

What's the best-kept secret in health care for Alzheimer's patients? Surprise! It's adult day care centers. Using a center can be nearly magical—both for your loved one and for you as the primary caregiver.

For the person with AD, a few hours at an adult day care center means a change of scenery, social interactions, mental stimulation, and something to look forward to. For the caregiver, it can be wonderful respite from the relentless grind of caregiving. As authors Nancy Mace and Peter Rabins say in their book *The 36-Hour Day*, "Taking time out, away from the care of an impaired person, is one of the single most important things that you can do."

Caregivers can rest, go to work, run errands, or just live their own lives while their loved ones are safe at a center. For AD patients living alone and for long-distance caregivers, adult day care represents a protective setting, companionship, and a safety net during a portion of the day.

Adult day care can ease the difficult transition from home care by a family member to institutionalized care by long-term facility professionals. Many experts believe adult day care may even delay or permanently eliminate the need for institutionalization (except for late-stage AD). The caregiver can keep going because she can look forward to a regular break. AD patients, especially those living alone, can often maintain their independence longer.

According to the National Adult Day Services Association,

nearly 78 percent of adult day centers are operated as nonprofit organizations, usually by local government, senior centers, medical centers, and community and religious groups. Facilities range from full-service "mini-resorts" to the proverbial church basement. Most centers are open during weekday business hours and some offer transportation services. Only a few have weekend or evening programs, and none offer overnight stays.

There are two basic types of adult day care. One is primarily social while the other is focused on medical/health services. Social centers provide structured, comprehensive, and individualized programs, meals, recreational and educational activities, and a few health services. Medically focused centers are staffed by skilled medical personnel to handle later-stage AD problems and other serious health conditions.

Daily fees are less than home health aide visits and much less than the cost of skilled nursing. The average national cost is fifty-six dollars per day. Costs are based on activities and the level of skilled care needed. Centers may offer fees on a sliding scale based on clients' income or personal circumstances. Some long-term care insurance plans and some states' Medicaid waiver programs offer partial reimbursement of costs.

The following Best Questions will help you find a top-quality adult day care center if you live in an area where you can choose from several different ones. Even if you have few choices, these questions can still help with your peace of mind, by helping you confirm that your loved one will be in good hands. There are two separate question lists here. The first list is what to ask the center's director or staff before enrollment. The second question list is what to ask yourself after you have toured the center in order to evaluate what you've observed with your own two eyes.

>>>THE 10 BEST QUESTIONS
to Find Quality Adult Day Care for Alzheimer's Patients

1. Is the center licensed by the state and accredited with a national day care accreditation program? How long has it been in operation? Who owns and runs the center?

Not all states license and regulate adult day care centers. Check with your local Area Agencies on Aging (in the telephone book), the Eldercare Locator (www.eldercare.gov), and the Better Business Bureau (www.bbb.org).

Because the demand for adult day care services is relatively new and growing rapidly, there are few standards for excellence, regulations, or inspections to help you judge quality. As a result, there may be a great deal of difference between individual centers.

Ask to see the center's license and latest inspection report. Knowing how long the center has been in operation and if it operates as a nonprofit or for-profit organization will help you assess its reliability and value. If you have choices, visit several centers near you (or near the AD patient) and talk with the staff and other families who use the center.

2. What are the qualifications, experience, and length of service of the center's administrative staff and aides?

Many centers have limited budgets and must rely heavily on part-time workers or volunteers. As a result, there is often high turnover among employees, low expectations for quality staff performance, and few hiring requirements.

However, you still want to be assured that the staff has been fully checked, including background checks for past criminal records. A policy of regular staff evaluations indicates that employees are being held accountable for meeting performance standards.

Ask what the client-to-employee ratio is to ensure there are

enough workers to offer creative activities and one-on-one attention as needed. Expect higher levels of staff professionalism and
medical expertise in a medically oriented center.

Here are more follow-up questions to clarify the staff's credentials. Do staff members have dementia-specific training? Does the
center have a physician, nurse, or licensed health care professional
on the premises or on call? If the center uses volunteers, are they
adequately trained and supervised?

3. How convenient is the center and its operating hours for me/my loved one? Can we make arrangements for transportation?

The convenience of a center is a very important consideration, especially for frequent or daily use. If you work or have other commit-
ments, its operating hours can be crucial, as well as the availability
of transportation.

It's equally important, though, not to choose an adult day care
center solely based on its convenience or cost. Overall, quality is
more important than location.

4. What services are available? What is a typical day like?

The ideal day care facility for Alzheimer's patients is specifically
designed for them, including their own segregated area away from
other seniors using the facility.

Ask if this center offers mainly social or medical services to
match your needs. Social centers should highlight games, mental
activities, field trips, educational programs, socializing, and exercise classes. Look for therapeutic activities that encourage thinking
abilities and help to improve memory, strength, mobility, and dex-
terity. Some locations even offer hairstyling services, counseling,
and support groups.

Medically focused centers offer assessments, rehabilitation,
blood pressure checks, and medication reminders. If your loved one

> **THE QUESTION DOCTOR SAYS:**
>
> A great adult day care center, regardless of size or cost, is the one that treats you and your loved ones as unique individuals and greets you by name with a warm welcome.

requires more medical care, choose a facility staffed by skilled nurses, social workers, and physical therapists with a high staff-to-participant ratio.

Be practical, too. As Clare Absher, an experienced geriatric nurse in North Carolina says, "We all want the place to look like a cruise ship so we feel better about leaving our loved one there. But the physical environment is really not that significant. A homey rambler or ranch-style building with good nursing care and only a TV can be just as good for the person with Alzheimer's."

5. Will the center evaluate my/my loved one's individualized needs and develop an activities plan?

Within reason, you want to choose a facility that will work closely with your loved one to tailor its programs to her specific needs, interests, and cognitive level. If the center does perform client evaluations, ask how it will be done, if you will have access to the results, and how often it will be repeated.

Other smart follow-up questions include, "Are all people required to participate at all times?" Will there be any progress reports?" "How will I know about my loved one's day and what's happening in the center (such as video webcams for remote monitoring)?" "Will the staff inform me on a daily basis about my loved one's well-being and any problems she had today?"

6. How does the center manage Alzheimer's problem behaviors, including wandering, aggression, improper sexual advances, incontinence, depression, and withdrawal?

The best answer to this Best Question includes a description of the special training that the staff has received in coping with Alzheimer's patients' behaviors. Even if you or your loved one doesn't display any of these bad behaviors, you still don't want to be exposed to an overabundance of them in others because they are being ignored or mishandled.

Ask about the center's polices on disciplinary methods and if food is ever used as a punishment or reward. Make sure that an occasional incident of incontinence isn't grounds for punishment or exclusion from the center. If possible, visit during a late afternoon when AD patients are likely to be "sundowning" (agitation or restlessness) to see for yourself how well the staff routinely handles people with late-day confusion and problem behaviors.

7. What precautions are in place to ensure safety and to deal with emergencies?

Safety and security are paramount concerns.

Look for safe wandering areas indoors and outside (such as a secured courtyard or garden), well-marked hallways, quality lighting, privacy areas, accessible bathrooms, and a nurturing, comfortable ambiance.

Ask about fire and safety policies, including a posted fire escape route, fire extinguisher, regular safety inspections, a sprinkler system, and a written emergency preparedness plan. Inquire about specialized staff training to help disabled or confused people escape during an emergency.

Find out if the staff has been trained in first aid and CPR at a minimum. Ask if a doctor is always on call and what are the procedures when there is an accident on the premises.

8. Does the center provide meals or snacks? If so, what are the center's nutrition policies? How will my loved one's nutritional needs be met?

Ask if you can sample a meal or a snack yourself. Ideally, return another time unannounced to try the food again.

Request to see a typical menu or food plan. Ask how the center will accommodate special dietary needs, such as a culturally specific menu or food allergies. Inquire about any extra costs for certain foods or special menus.

9. Are the costs, eligibility, admission, and discharge standards spelled out in writing and clarified in advance?

Since Alzheimer's disease is a progressive disorder, you want to know in advance how the center will deal with someone's worsening condition. Most centers exclude late-stage AD patients with severe problem behaviors. Get the specifics now.

In addition to daily charges, ask if you must pay anything in advance. If so, ask about the center's policies for paying during absences, holidays, and illnesses. Discuss transportation costs and any possible hidden fees (craft supplies, field trips, etc.). Inquire about fees for initiation, deposits, late arrivals, or late pickups. Do you have to pay for any programs booked but not actually attended?

10. What are the names and contact details for three clients/AD caregivers whom I can talk to?

This request is common practice and the center should already have made prearrangements for client referrals. When you talk to the referrals, ask them for the center's strengths, weaknesses, and past performance in handling problems ranging from daily difficult AD behaviors to medical emergencies. Focus especially on their impression of the staff, including qualifications, turnover, and their responsiveness to individuals' needs and interests.

❯ The Magic Question

What do you do to help your staff and volunteers avoid burnout? How do you reward your best employees?

Staffing and retaining personnel at an Alzheimer's day care center can be really tough. The centers often have small budgets and may rely on unpaid volunteers.

Even if the majority of center workers are unpaid volunteers, understanding how well this center treats its people will give you a glimpse into the care you can expect for your loved one. If you are paying for skilled care at a medically based center, you should have higher expectations for a structured personnel system, including employee benefits, specialized training, and adequate time off.

THE 10 BEST QUESTIONS TO ASK YOURSELF AFTER TOURING AN ADULT DAY CARE CENTER

1. **Was the staff warm and friendly?**
   An outgoing and pleasant staff without personality clashes among themselves is more likely to interact well with you and your loved one.

2. **How well did the staff handle any problem behaviors that I witnessed?**
   Easy competence indicates specialized Alzheimer's training, solid experience, or both.

3. **Did the Alzheimer's patients look calm, safe, and busy?**
   Patient happiness is not always within the staff's control, but you can spot patterns in

patients' facial expressions, levels of sociability, and the center's general ambiance or "personality."

4. **Was there a place to isolate sick, aggressive, or agitated people?**
   Having a "holding room" protects others at the center from illness or physical harm.

5. **Was the facility clean, did it feel inviting, and was it free of unpleasant odors?**
   Use your senses to see, touch, and smell the facility for potential problems. Look for small touches like furniture groupings that encourage interaction.

6. **How elderly friendly were the furniture and public areas?**
   Adult day care should be carefully geared toward the special needs of older or disabled people, including wheelchair ramps, bathroom grab bars, sturdy sofas, and well-lit rooms.

7. **Did someone on the staff take a personal interest in me and my loved one?**
   You want a center that sees each person as a unique individual and not just someone else to "babysit" for the day.

8. **Do I agree with the center's policies and practices for handling Alzheimer's behavior problems?**
   Verify that this center shares your personal beliefs about discipline problems like wandering or aggression. You don't want your loved one to come home with a black eye (or deliver one either)!

9. **How well were my 10 Best Questions answered?**
   Patience with your questions and a willingness to educate you are positive signs of a well-run facility.

10. **Are the Alzheimer's patients and regular clients kept separated?**
    Integrating AD patients with others receives mixed reviews among experts, but most agree AD patients with advanced symptoms should not mingle with other center clients, if they are even admitted at all.

The Magic Question

Would I want to spend time here?
Ideally, the environment should be pleasant, the activities fun and engaging, and the services and staff ones that you would freely choose for yourself.

CONCLUSION

Evaluate the staff with the same thoroughness as you do the environment of the facility. Observe how staffers treat the most difficult Alzheimer's patients. Ironically, the same evaluation criteria to choose a child-care facility applies to adult day care as well, including individualized attention and plans, clearly written policies on acceptable behaviors and costs, guarantees for pleasant surroundings, and an emphasis on safety, education, medical issues, socializing, and having fun.

Even if you must travel a little farther, it's worth finding a competent and reliable adult day care center so you can enjoy your time off worry free. Both the caregiver and AD patient have everything to gain from the break away from each other. Adult day care can be an absolute God-sent lifesaver for overwhelmed and stressed-out caregivers.

As *Elder Rage* author Jacqueline Marcell says, "Day care is so valuable for caregivers because when Alzheimer's patients are kept active during the day, they sleep better at night."

THE 10 BEST RESOURCES

American Association of Homes and Services for the Aging, "Excellence in Alzheimer's and Dementia Care" www.aahsa.org/pubs_resources/futureage/best_practices/documents/BP_V2N1_JAN_FEB03/Excellence_Alzheimers_Dementia_v2n1.pdf.

Eldercare Locator. "Fact Sheets: Adult Day Care." www.eldercare.gov/Eldercare/Public/resources/fact_sheets/adult_day.asp.

Helpguide. "Adult Day Care Centers: A Guide to Options and Selecting the Best Center for Your Needs." www.helpguide.org/elder/adult_day_care_centers.htm.

Linderman, David. *Alzheimer's Day Care: A Basic Guide.* New York: Hemisphere Publishing, 1991.

Mace, Nancy, and Peter Rabins. "Getting Outside Help." In *The 36-Hour Day: A Family Guide to Caring for Persons with Alzheimer Disease, Related Dementing Illnesses, and Memory Loss in Later Life,* 4th ed. Baltimore, Md.: The Johns Hopkins University Press, 2006.

MetLife. "Adult Day Centers." www.metlife.com/FileAssets/MMI/MMI SYCAdultDayCenters2007.pdf.

National Adult Day Services Association, "Adult Day Services: Overview and Facts." www.nadsa.org/adsfacts/default.asp.

National Adult Day Services Association. "Selecting Quality Providers," www.nadsa.org/quality_providers/default.asp.

National Adult Day Services Association. *Standards and Guidelines for Adult Day Services.* Seattle, Wash.: National Adult Day Services Association, 1997.

National Association of Area Agencies on Aging. "Eldercare Locator." Provides connections to local community-based services. www.n4a.org/locator.

CHAPTER 14: THE 10 BEST QUESTIONS
to Hire a Top Home Health
Care Agency

No man, not even a doctor, ever gives any other
definition of what a nurse should be than this,
"devoted and obedient."

—Florence Nightingale

Home care agencies and home care aides provide critical
health care services and assistance with the Activities of
Daily Living (ADLs) for Alzheimer's patients living in
their own homes, especially for advanced AD. Both the AD patient
and the caregiver can benefit from in-home services. Having paid
in-home help extends the amount of time your loved one can remain at home before relocating to a long-term care facility. As the
caregiver, you may be at your wit's end trying to manage your loved
one's increasingly difficult behaviors or medical problems.

There are two general types of home health care services—
skilled care and nonskilled care. Skilled care is performed by licensed professionals, such as registered nurses (RNs), licensed
practical nurses (LPNs), physical therapists, social workers, speech
pathologists, occupational therapists, and dietitians. For example,
skilled nurses provide the initial consultation and monitor medications. Nonskilled care, including home health aides, personal aides,
homemakers, and companions, help with the Activities of Daily
Living under the guidance of a professional. There are also parapro-
fessionals called certified nurses aides who assist with ADLs but
also can perform simple medical tasks, like taking blood pressure
and pulses, after passing a certifying exam.

Once you've identified home care agencies in your area, you'll want to know more about each agency, its services, and especially about the strangers who will be entering your home and providing care for your loved one.

Ask the following Best Questions when you are interviewing prospective agencies. Take notes and compare agencies before you make your decision.

>>> THE 10 BEST QUESTIONS
to Hire a Top Home Health Care Agency

1. Is your agency licensed, bonded, and accredited?

Unfortunately, not all states require that agencies have licenses to operate. Check the National Association for Home Care and Hospice Web site (www.nahc.org/Consumer/resources.html) for providers in your state. In states with requirements, licensure and bonding are your assurance that an agency meets the minimum standards set by the state.

Accreditation by a nationally recognized organization is the gold standard to look for. This is because agencies are not required to be accredited, so the best ones have gone this extra step for quality and recognition. The top accrediting organizations include The Joint Commission (www.jointcommission.org), Accreditation Commission for Health Care (www.ache.org) Community Health Accreditation Program (www.chapinc.org/aboutus.htm), and Home Care University (www.nahc.org/HCU/home.html).

Dale Johnson, an executive director at The Joint Commission, says, "You want an agency that has sought and been accredited by an outside organization."

Ask if the agency is Medicare certified. A Medicare-certified agency must meet federal minimum requirements for patient care and management.

2. How long has this agency been in business and operating in this community, region, or state? Who owns it and where are they headquartered?

The longer the agency has been in business, the better for you. They will have had time to hire solid employees, work out internal processes, learn from their mistakes (you hope), and learn how to manage problems.

Ownership of home care agencies ranges from megacorporations headquartered overseas to small family-owned, homegrown firms. Some nonprofit agencies are sponsored through community or religious organizations.

In general, large corporations can offer more services, while smaller companies offer more personalized care. Look for managers who have health-related backgrounds, such as nurses or therapists, and especially managers who are savvy about Alzheimer's patients' behavioral problems and medical conditions. Ask if this agency has a Web site or written literature that discloses its funding sources, annual report, and company background.

3. How does your agency select and train your employees?

This is a critical and complex Best Question. Ultimately the quality of care your loved one receives is dependent on the quality of the aides sent from this agency.

To make sure, ask these additional important questions:

- What specific training in Alzheimer's care do you provide to your staff?
- Describe this training in detail (topics, length of training, minimal pass level, etc.).
- Do I have your assurances that the aide who will be assigned to us has this training in AD?

- How do you support and protect your workers?
- Do you have written personnel policies and performance standards, benefits packages, and malpractice insurance for your aides?
- Are aides individually licensed and bonded?
- What is your staff turnover rate?
- How do you alleviate job burnout, especially for aides working with AD patients?

Don't forget to ask the last question. Aide burnout can result in elder abuse or neglect, just as it can with family caregiver burnout. Home care aides are typically underpaid and overworked, so burnout can be a real problem.

4. Do you provide a home evaluation prior to the first service visit? If so, how comprehensive is this evaluation? Who performs this evaluation?

The best answer is, Yes, there is a free comprehensive home evaluation done by a registered nurse (RN) or therapist. A home evaluation is comprehensive if it includes consultation with the patient's doctors and family members and is tailored to consider the needs of an Alzheimer's patient at the same stage as your loved one.

Look for the agency to provide you with a copy of a Patient Bill of Rights and a statement to protect confidentiality. Also look for a patient-centered focus, where the nurse seems to anticipate your needs and concerns before you express them.

5. Does your agency develop a written plan of care for your AD patients? If so, are the caregiver, family, and patient involved in this process?

Your agreement with this agency should require them to provide a written, individualized plan of care at the outset of the contract.

The trick is making sure that this plan will be updated periodically to show actual, specific goals accomplished and to match care adjustments with your loved one's changing needs. Ask how often the plan is updated, if caregivers are involved, and if you'll receive a copy.

This is also a good time to ask questions about the individual who will be coming to your home. The agency may not have chosen a specific person yet, but ask these general questions:

- How do you match your aides/skilled caregivers to clients' needs and personalities?
- Will your agency try to assign us the same aide/caregiver consistently?
- Do we get to meet and talk with this person in advance?
- Is a short trial period possible prior to the actual contracted time?
- What happens if we want to change aides? What is your policy?

6. Who will supervise the quality of care for my loved one? How can I reach this person?

The supervisor should be a professional manager or nurse. You want the agency's total assurance there will be a responsible, accountable supervisor to oversee the quality of care for your loved one. Ask if the agency sends supervisors to your home for regular evaluations and if there's a charge for these visits.

7. How is the quality of care and services monitored over time? How does your agency resolve problems and client complaints?

Routine visits to the home by the supervisor should be the norm, not the exception. Get the details and any other ways the agency ensures quality care.

THE QUESTION DOCTOR SAYS:

This "who" question is really critical. Be sure you get the supervisor's name, phone number, and e-mail address.

Don't settle for just a vague position title and a main office phone number. Ask what hours and days this person is available to you. You want to know exactly who will come to your loved one's home and make things right if there are problems.

How a company deals with problems and complaints separates the good agencies from the great ones. If you get a vague response to this question, ask for a description of a past problem (preferably with an Alzheimer's patient) and what specifically the agency did to resolve the situation.

Make sure you know whom to call for problems if it's not the regular supervisor.

8. How do you deal with medical emergencies in the home?

You want to hear that this agency has routine, detailed procedures for handling medical emergencies. Even the unskilled aides should be trained in first aid and CPR techniques at a minimum. A good follow-up question is to ask if there is a nursing supervisor on call twenty-four hours a day.

9. What are your costs and a description of your services?

Request a detailed, written explanation of this agency's fees, services, and eligibility requirements. Make sure you understand what level of care (skilled or nonskilled) you are paying for and the daily or hourly rates.

Follow-up questions on costs include:

- Is there a fee for the initial assessment?
- Is there a minimum number of hours I must contract for?
- Is there a sliding fee scale?
- How will I be billed, how frequently, and will the bills be itemized?
- Are there any additional costs, such as the purchase or rental of special equipment, not readily obvious in this contract?
- Will I be charged extra fees for supervisory visits, running errands, or transportation services?
- Are there different fees for holidays, weekends, and overnight stays?
- What arrangements are available if my reimbursement sources become exhausted?

Medicare will pay for home care for beneficiaries with Alzheimer's disease under certain conditions, but custodial needs (ADLs) are rarely covered. Check with your managed care provider and private insurance plans to learn about coverage in your case.

10. Please provide me with a list of three previous clients whom I can contact for referrals.

Ask for a list of previous clients whom you can call for referrals, preferably people with similar situations to yours. These references might include doctors, nurses, caregivers, or community leaders who know this agency's services well.

When you call, ask each referral the following questions:

- Do you frequently refer others to this agency? Why or why not?
- What experiences, if any, with this agency were unpleasant? Why?

- How responsive were they to dealing with your questions and problems?
- What specifically did they do to fix problems?
- Did a nurse or supervisor conduct follow-up visits? How comprehensive were they? How frequent?
- Would you hire this agency again? Why or why not?
- Do you have a contractual relationship with this agency as a paid referral? If so, do you require that it meets special standards for quality care?

❯ The Magic Question

Does your agency conduct full criminal background checks on all your prospective workers?

Although most states require agencies to perform criminal background checks, regulations vary from state to state. Check with your local Agency on Aging. A full criminal background check should include searches of the following records: arrests, court orders, driving records, criminal history, sex offender status, and bankruptcy checks. Make sure that new employees are not allowed to work in your home before their background check has been completed.

Even if the employees' histories are clean, you still want to make sure that the agency is holding them accountable for their current conduct, too. So ask these follow-up questions:

- Do you conduct routine, random drug checks on your current workers?
- What are your policies for discipline and dismissal?
- How many employees have been fired for any reason in the last two years?

One rotten apple can spoil even the best home care agency. Doing your homework is your best guarantee that your loved one won't be injured or neglected and that your beloved grandmother's diamond brooch won't be sold for drug money.

CONCLUSION

Half of all family caregivers also work outside the home. Caring for a person with later-stage AD is physically and emotionally draining. No wonder caregivers often need help. Hiring a home care agency to send skilled or unskilled help into your home is a less expensive and transitional alternative to nursing home care. But most family caregivers are uneasy at the prospect of having a stranger come into their home to work hands-on with their loved one. This is often both an emotional and practical decision for weary caregivers.

Finding a reliable home health agency may seem like a formidable task at first. There are thousands of public and private organizations nationwide, with new ones opening up every day. Experienced geriatric nurse and consultant Clare Absher advises, "If you don't get a level of care with a nurse coming out initially to explain their services and match the caregiving you need, then move on to the next agency."

You need a combination of close scrutiny, a skeptical outlook, and these Best Questions to avoid being disappointed or ripped off. Keep in mind that regardless of the agency's reputation and how much you like a certain aide or nurse, government regulations and strict industry standards haven't kept up with an exploding demand for home health care services. With so few safeguards in place, you must stay vigilant.

THE 10 BEST RESOURCES

Administration on Aging. "Home Health Care: A Guide for Families." www.aoa.gov/press/prodsmats/fact/pdf/HomeHealthFS.pdf.

American Association of Homes and Services for the Aging. "Homes and Services Directory." www.aahsa.org/consumer_info/homes_svcs_directory/default.asp.

American Medical Association. *American Medical Association Guide to Home Caregiving.* New York: John Wiley and Sons, 2001.

Centers for Medicare and Medicaid Services. "Medicare and Home Health Care." www.medicare.gov/publications/pubs/pdf/10969.pdf.

Community Health Accreditation Program. "CHAP Accredited Agencies." Accreditation database searchable by agency name or state. www.chapapps.org/search.

Joint Commission. "Helping You Choose Quality Home Care and Hospice Services." www.jointcommission.org/GeneralPublic/Choices/hc_ome.htm.

Mayo Clinic. "Home Care Services: Questions to Ask." www.mayoclinic.com/print/home-care-services/HO00084.

Medicare. "Home Health Compare." Searchable database on all Medicare-certified home health agencies in the United States. www.medicare.gov/HHCompare/Home.asp?version=default&browser=IE%7C7%7CWinXP&language=English&defaultstatus=0&pagelist=Home&CookiesEnabledStatus=True.

MetLife. "Understanding Home Care Agency Options." www.metlife.com/WPSAssets/17497016641050493636V1FUnderstanding%20Home%20Care%20Agency%20Options%203-03.pdf.

National Association for Home Care and Hospice. "How to Choose a Home Care Provider." www.nahc.org/Consumer/contents.html.

CHAPTER 15: THE 10 BEST QUESTIONS

to Choose a Long-Term Care Facility
for an Alzheimer's Resident

Always be nice to your children because they are the ones
who will choose your rest home.

—Phyllis Diller

No matter how well you have cared for your loved one
with Alzheimer's disease at home, the day will come
when you simply can no longer provide the level of care
she needs. You will be faced with choosing a long-term care residential facility. For most caregivers, this becomes a necessary step
at the point that their loved one has developed severe behavioral
problems, advanced memory impairment, or other serious medical
conditions.

This may be one of the most painful decisions you ever make.
You may be racked by guilt because you promised your loved one
never to "put her away." You may face stiff resistance from your
loved one or from other family members and friends who criticize
you from the sidelines without fully comprehending the enormity
of caregiving for advanced AD.

Your options for long-term residential care are determined in
part by your loved one's AD stage. Most assisted living residences
don't have the round-the-clock medical staff needed to care for late-
stage AD patients, with the exception of assisted living homes with
special Alzheimer's units.

In smaller communities, there may be licensed residential care
homes called adult family homes or group homes. These provide
room and board and assistance with daily living activities. Although these board and care homes can be excellent, some states

don't require licensing, which means you need to choose one very carefully.

Nursing homes are similar to hospitals because of their emphasis on skilled nursing care. They provide medical professionals and support staff twenty-four hours a day and routinely provide assistance with the activities of daily living (bathing, dressing, toileting, etc.). In comparison, the residents in assisted living facilities generally have a more independent lifestyle.

Laura Nichols, the director of the Northern Virginia Long-Term Care Ombudsman Program, which deals with complaints about long-term care facilities, advises, "When you are looking for a facility, *research* it, don't just go to the one that is closest."

The following 10 Best Questions will help you choose any type of long-term care facility wisely for your loved one with Alzheimer's disease. Be sure to check out more than one facility, visit each one several times, and use at least one of the quality search tools/Web sites referenced at the end of this chapter. Location and cost are important but are not the only decision factors.

THE QUESTION DOCTOR SAYS:

Don't be swayed by guilt or criticism. You must make the decision based on what's best for the health and safety of your loved one, you, and your family. Most people dislike and fear nursing homes, often imaging the worst cases of loneliness, abandonment, neglect, and abuse.

Good homes are hard to find, but if you use your common sense, keep your eyes wide open on the tour, and ask lots of questions, you'll make the best-informed decision possible.

The best facilities often have long waiting lists, so start your search early. Call first before visiting facilities and ask about bed availability and if the facility accepts your insurance or Medicare. If they say yes, you'll be ready to ask this chapter's Best Questions and your own questions as well.

〉〉〉THE 10 BEST QUESTIONS
to Choose a Long-Term Care Facility for an Alzheimer's Resident

1. Is this facility accredited by The Joint Commission? Is it licensed in this state? Is it Medicare and Medicaid certified?

Accreditation matters. Being accredited means the facility has voluntarily chosen to be evaluated and has met the most rigorous quality standards in the industry as set by The Joint Commission. Look for The Joint Commission Gold Seal of Approval when selecting your nursing home as a clear sign of compliance with these most stringent standards.

However, The Joint Commission's executive director for the long-term care accreditation, Dale Johnson, warns, "Just because you see a gold seal on the front door, that doesn't mean that it's been accredited in the Alzheimer's unit." Also ask specifically about the AD unit.

The level of accreditation matters too. For example, some facilities may claim to be accredited, but they actually have only a provisional or conditional accreditation due to serious deficiencies. Ask about the facility's specific level as explained below.

- **Accreditation.** Shows full compliance with all standards.
- **Preliminary accreditation.** Shows compliance but official accreditation status is pending more information.
- **Provisional accreditation.** Fails to address all required improvements on a timely basis.
- **Conditional accreditation.** Fails to be in substantial compliance with standards.
- **Preliminary denial of accreditation.** Fails in compliance and standards beyond established thresholds.

- **Denial of accreditation.** Fails to meet requirements or re-solve a previous conditional status.

Find out if this facility is licensed by your state or locality. If so, it will have met certain standards set by your state or local government. Each state is responsible for inspecting nursing homes every nine to fifteen months for license renewal. These reports are available to the public.

Make sure the facility is Medicare and Medicaid certified as a minimum of acceptable quality. This means the facility has passed an inspection by the state survey agency. Keep in mind that being certified is not the same as being accredited.

As a follow-up question, ask, "Are there any unresolved state compliance, licensing, or health care issues with this residence?" A 2003 report by Consumers Union identified by state the 10 percent of nursing homes whose inspection reports raised serious questions about the quality of care given to residents.

2. How convenient is this facility to the primary caregiver or other family members or friends who plan regular visits?

Location also matters. You want a top-rated care facility, but it's also smart to choose one that is fairly accessible for the people who will be visiting the AD resident.

Visitors matter—a lot—because they increase the likelihood that your loved one will get better attention and more consistent care. If the facility's staff realizes an outside pair of eyes and ears are overseeing their interactions with a resident, that resident can benefit in many ways.

Even when your loved one no longer recognizes you or other family or friends, continue to visit him on a regular (and unannounced) basis so you can be his personal watchdog against staff neglect or abuse.

3. Does this facility have a dedicated Alzheimer's unit? If so, does the staff receive special training in dealing with AD residents?

Increasingly, nursing homes and assisted living residences are establishing special units for people with moderate to severe Alzheimer's disease. Special care units should provide active therapy and behavioral management for AD residents who wander and are difficult to manage. Ask about bed availability, eligibility requirements, and additional costs for this unit.

Experienced geriatric nurse Clare Absher believes, "If you have a choice, the most important consideration is whether or not they really have a designated area for Alzheimer's patients and not just a section where they've put up a sign. The way to tell is to ask about the staff's special, ongoing training in Alzheimer's care. For example, AD patients are often afraid of water, but someone with special training will know how to bathe them."

Ask to see the facility's written statement of its "philosophy of the unit" and look for a therapeutic, resident-centered approach to care. Also ask, "Will my loved one have to be transferred to another unit or building wing later as his condition worsens?" and "How do you handle difficult behavior problems?" Compare meals served here with the main dining hall for quality and variety.

Experts recommend that staffing ratios should be one staff person to five residents for daytime shifts and at least a one to nine ratio for overnight/weekend shifts. Ask how staff members deal with AD residents' sundowners (late-afternoon agitation or restlessness) or sleeplessness and about the use of chemical or physical restraints for AD residents. Inquire if a geriatric psychiatrist experienced with AD is affiliated with the unit. Ask, "Does the psychiatrist evaluate residents' psychoactive medications on a routine basis? Is the family *always* notified?"

4. What are the staff's training, qualifications, and turnover rates? Do you do criminal background checks on all your employees?

The staff's size, qualifications, specialized training, and attitude toward the residents is one of the most critical variables to consider.

Most facilities are understaffed, so you want to assess how each facility copes with this unfortunate reality. Get the specifics on the exact credentials, certifications, and AD training for the direct care staff.

Ask these additional questions: "What is the ratio of hands-on workers to residents with AD?" (Ask it this way so janitorial staff, etc., can't be counted.) "How extensive are their criminal background checks (national versus local sources)?" "Are new employees allowed to work before their background checks are completed?" "Do you do routine, unannounced drug tests on your employees?" "If not, how can you assure me that my loved one is in safe hands?" "Has anyone on staff been formally accused of abuse or neglect?" "If so, what have you done about the complaint?" "Does the direct care staff speak English (or your native language) clearly?" "How consistent are the aides' assignments?" (to assess if staffers can get to know residents as individuals).

5. What are typical menus for Alzheimer's residents? How will I know my loved one is receiving proper nutrition and hydration?

Look at the menus for at least one month and eat in the dining hall yourself several times. Is the food tasty, nutritious, adequate, varied, and attractively served in a pleasant dining atmosphere? Ask if meals are prepared on premises or transported from another location.

Can menus, eating times, and eating locations be modified as needed? Does a nutritionist or dietitian review the meals and special diets? If so, how often?

How many meals and snacks are provided each day in the package price? Are nutritious snacks available all day including after hours? Are serving locations flexible (trays served in residents' rooms, for example), and if so, at what additional cost? Can the kitchen accommodate special dietary needs and religious and ethnic preferences? Are there special holiday meals?

Be sure to ask about how the staff handles AD residents who refuse to eat. When eating is a problem, at what point is the family notified? The best menus in the world won't matter if someone isn't making sure your loved one eats properly.

Request a tour of the main kitchen. Look for well-washed utensils, clean cooking surfaces, pleasant smells, and a well-organized layout.

6. How does the facility handle grievances and problems? Are there written policies on residents' rights and responsibilities?

Most caregivers never think to ask about the facility's policies and procedures for handing complaints until they have one. Most assuredly, over time you will encounter problems, so find out now how this facility will resolve them. Written, formal procedures and policies are a good sign, but you also want proof that they aren't just giving it lip service.

Here are more questions to hold their feet to the fire. How are grievances handled by the administration or management? By the staff? What happens if a resident or family member does not agree with the residence's care plan? Is there a formal appeals process? If so, what typically happens during an appeal?

If a resident is unhappy with some aspect of the facility, how are his complaints handled? What is the protocol for notifying family members about problems, conditions, or concerns? What role, if any, does the family council play in the grievance/appeals process?

What's an example of a past grievance? How was it handled by staff administration or the nursing staff? Who owns this facility and do they ever become involved with grievances? Who is the main contact person for dealing with problems? Finally, ask about their long-term care ombudsman program and contact information.

7. What are the facility's policies on outsiders' visits? Is there an active family council in place? If so, how does the facility deal with the council's concerns?

Find out if family members and friends are allowed and encouraged to visit often with liberal visiting hours. This policy should include welcoming outsiders into the dining hall and allowing them to be with sick loved ones during off hours. A liberal visitation policy indicates the recognition of residents' social and emotional needs and that the facility isn't trying to hide something. Make sure to visit the facility unannounced several times at mealtimes, at night, and on the weekends.

There should be a **family council** (also called a **resident conference**) composed of family members and caregivers who meet regularly to discuss quality, safety, and lifestyle issues for their loved ones. Ask, "Who runs the council? What happens to the council's suggestions and grievances? What is their track record for successfully initiating changes?"

Find out if there is a support group affiliated with this facility just for families and caregivers of AD residents, which is another good sign of family-friendly policies. Ask if there are other outsiders allowed, such as a programs bringing in companion animals, music therapy, or community volunteers. Residents who were separated from their pets to enter a facility are at particular risk for social isolation and withdrawal.

8. What are your policies and procedures for after-hours care, medical emergencies, and handling medications?

Expect to see clear, written procedures and a statement of residents' rights for responding to medical emergencies, especially during overnight hours and on weekends. After-hours care and coverage is critical. Many medical emergencies occur during off hours when facilities are typically understaffed. The very time of day that your loved one may be the most vulnerable is exactly the point of lowest staff coverage.

Here are more questions about after-hours care. Are resident checks made routinely during the night? If so, how frequently? Is the front desk manned twenty-four hours a day? What are the protocols for checking on residents who have not been seen for more than twelve hours? For notifying families? How many staff are *on-site* at night and how reliable is their communication system for dealing with problems?

Here are more related questions. What are the credentials of the primary care physicians used by the facility and what services do they provide? How often do doctors visit for routine checkups? What hospital affiliations do the doctors and nurses have? How close is the nearest hospital? What training has the direct care staff received to handle problems and emergencies? Under what circumstances does the facility call 911? Call the family? Call the doctor? Who decides and what are his medical credentials?

How are medications administrated? By whom and what is their medical training? What safeguards ensure that residents get their correct medications and dosages? Who supervises and reviews the medication procedures? What are their qualifications?

Are there additional fees for assistance or can residents administer their own medications? How are medications stored for safety?

Do residents have to buy medications in house or can they use their current pharmacy? What is this facility's medication error rate?

9. Has this facility created pleasant living spaces for its AD residents that are clean, autonomous, safe, and secure?

AD significantly changes how people interpret what they see, hear, taste, feel, and smell. Overstimulation or understimulation of the senses can cause confusion and agitation. An environment that is well suited to AD residents requires special attention and individualized care.

Ombudsman director Laura Nichols says, "Don't be fooled by the expensive decor. This does not equate to better care." Look beyond the public areas and assess the residents' rooms for comfort and safety features, such as grab bars in the bathroom, adequate lighting and temperature controls, and colored-coded passageways. Check out the shower room and bathing schedules.

Ask about the facility's security measures to protect residents' personal possessions and cash, safe areas for wanderers, and the whole building's security system. Be sure to ask about the facility's emergency plans to assist AD and immobile residents in case of fire or other catastrophic emergency, such as a flood, tornado, or earthquake.

10. What are the costs for initial deposit, monthly fees, additional fees, and the terms of the contract? Are we provided with a written plan of care?

Costs depend on the level of care required. In general, assisted living residences, which require less staff, are cheaper than nursing homes. Nursing home fees range from $2,500 to $7,000 and more per month. A 2008 study by Genworth Financial found the average annual cost of a private room in a nursing home was $76,460, or

$209 per day, while the national average for assisted living facilities was $36,090 annually.

Medicare may cover some costs of nursing home care under some certain conditions. See the details in Medicare's booklet "Guide to Choosing a Nursing Home," or contact your State Health Insurance Assistance Program (see the references at the end of the chapter).

Ask the facility these questions: Do you develop a written care plan for new residents, including provision for additional care needs as the AD worsens? If so, how does this process work and what exactly are the additional services and additional costs at each level of increased care? How often are residents reassessed? Who makes these decisions and what are their medical credentials?

Many facilities have specific fees for every additional service performed on a daily basis, such as assistance with eating, which can add up quickly. All additional fees should be clearly itemized and given to you in writing.

Make sure you understand fully all the details of the contract. Take it to a legal professional or a trusted friend for review if you have any questions or doubts not fully addressed in your meetings with the facility's staff.

Ask these questions, too: What type of payment does the facility accept? Private pay only? Medicaid? Medicare? Grants? Does the contract provide fully descriptive and detailed explanations of the facility's responsibilities for the care of residents? Details about which services are included in the monthly charge? Exact fees for initial assessment, admission, and deposit? Exact fees for routine additional services? The rights of residents, including their rights if the residency closes or goes bankrupt? Is there a maximum ceiling on costs? What happens when a private pay resident becomes Medicare eligible?

THE 10 BEST QUESTIONS WHEN TOURING A LONG-TERM CARE FACILITY

The Joint Commission's nursing home specialist, Dale Johnson, suggests, "The best way to know is to go visit yourself and observe. If you overhear the staff talking about so-and-so's mom or calling her by name, that's a different level of care than the staff who refers to 'the patient in bed A' or 'the person who loses his socks.' "

Don't fall for the glitzy tour pitch from the facility's director. During the tour, ask yourself these questions while you keep your eyes, ears, and nose on full alert. The following Best Questions have been adapted from AARP's warning signs for bad nursing homes.

1. Are there strong odors, particularly of urine or heavy disinfectant as a cover-up?
2. How clean is the facility? (Ask to see an occupied resident's room to judge janitorial care.)
3. Do you see the use of restraints, such as chair, bed, or wheelchair straps or vests, or bruises, welts, or cuts on the residents?
4. Are residents' needs for privacy treated with respect, such as undressing them in private?
5. Does the staff speak to the residents (or one another) rudely or disrespectfully? Do staffers know residents by name and as individuals? Are the staffers speaking in a language your loved one doesn't know?
6. Are calls for help answered promptly? Are there grab bars and other safety features?
7. Are residents' food trays full or only half eaten? Are staffers helping residents to eat?
8. Do residents look lonely, unhappy, inactive, or immobile? Are they clean, dressed, and groomed?
9. Are you greeted or acknowledged by staff members, or is your presence ignored or even resented?
10. Is there a wide discrepancy between how well decorated and brightly lit the lobby/common areas are compared to the residents' hallways and rooms?

Long-time caregiver and author Patricia Callone suggests, "I recommend making pop-in visits unannounced around mealtime to see if people have eaten their food and to check for cleanliness."

How frequently are costs increased (ask for the average from the last five years)? Is there any way to lock in lower prices with prepayments or other arrangements? How much advance notice is given for rate increases? What is the projected cost-of-living increase for the coming year?

Who is responsible for payment if the family's money runs out? Is there any kind of financial assistance for these cases?

❯ The Magic Question

What do you do to help your staff avoid burnout? How do you reward your best employees? Do you provide health care coverage to your staff?

Staffing and retaining an Alzheimer's unit is really tough. As a caregiver, you personally know that people with Alzheimer's are not always pleasant people to be around. The staff at these facilities need an occasional break to avoid burnout, just like primary caregivers do.

Understanding how well this facility treats its staff provides a window into the true level of care you can expect for your loved one. You want a facility that offers its staff good financial rewards, publicly recognizes excellent performance and dedication, and routinely offers stable assignments, training, and personal growth. If the staff has healthcare coverage, they will be more likely to stay home when they are sick and not infect the residents.

This is a Magic Question because it will probably catch many administrators by surprise. Listen for answers that include specific classes, opportunities for staff development or retreats, days off, and indicators that employees are commended rather than penalized for paying attention to their own needs, too.

Relatively happy staffers are more likely to have the patience,

> **AFTERWARD**
>
> Experienced ombudsman Laura Nichols offers these smart suggestions once you've chosen a long-term care facility:
>
> ❯ Know if there is a volunteer ombudsman and how to contact him.
>
> ❯ Learn who is the licensing agency for the facility, the contact person, and her number.
>
> ❯ Get a copy of the resident's basic information sheet to ensure all his emergency contact information is correct.
>
> ❯ Make sure you know who the main contact person is, her backup person, and contact details.
>
> ❯ Visit often and stay active in your loved one's life.

energy, and compassion they need to deal with difficult Alzheimer's residents and are less likely to include disgruntled workers, social misfits, or angry people who could take out their frustrations by neglecting or abusing your loved one.

CONCLUSION

Choosing a long-term care facility can be a very stressful yet necessary decision during your journey as the caregiver to a loved one with Alzheimer's disease. The patient's doctor may recommend this step, especially if the caregiver is a frail, elderly spouse or if the patient has progressed to late-stage AD.

Often, admission is for the benefit of the caregiver, to relieve her of the tremendous burden of home care. You as the caregiver should not feel guilt-ridden about this decision. You need to protect your own health and personal well-being.

Making this decision is not an exact science. Plan for enough in advance so that you can perform adequate research on your best options, go on tours, ask lots of questions, and learn about the facilities' quality and accreditation standards. There's also value in trusting your gut-level reactions and impressions from the tour.

Many advanced-stage AD patients require placement in a long-term care institution because the family caregiver is overwhelmed with stress and exhaustion to the point of collapse. Ideally, before this crisis point occurs, you will have done your homework to find the best long-term care that you can afford.

THE 10 BEST RESOURCES

Alzheimer's Association. "CareFinder." www.alz.org/carefinder/index.asp.

Centers for Medicare and Medicaid Services. "Guide to Choosing a Nursing Home." www.medicare.gov/Publications/Pubs/pdf/02174.pdf.

HealthGrades. "Compare Area Nursing Homes." www.healthgrades.com/consumer/index.cfm?fuseaction=mod&modtype=nhrc&modact=nhrc_search_form&tab_set=nursinghome&tv_lid=lnk_nh_top&tv_eng=home&tv_kw=nh_top.

Joint Commission, "Quality Check: Find a Health Care Organization." www.qualitycheck.org/consumer/searchQCR.aspx.

Medicare. "Long-Term Care Planning Tool." www.medicare.gov/LTCPlanning/Include/DataSection/Questions/SearchCriteria.asp?version=default&browser=IE%7C7%7CWinXP&language=English&defaultstatus=0&pagelist=Home.

Medicare. "Nursing Home Checklist." www.medicare.gov/nursing/checklist.pdf.

Medicare. "Nursing Home Compare." Provides details on all Medicare and Medicaid certified nursing homes. www.medicare.gov/nhcompare/home.asp.

Medicare. "Nursing Homes: Alternatives to Nursing Home Care." www.medicare.gov/nursing/alternatives.asp.

Medicare. "State Health Insurance Assistance Program (SHIP) Contact Information." www.medicare.gov/contacts/static/allStateContacts.asp.

National Long-Term Care Ombudsman Resource Center. "Ombudsmen (by State)." www.ltcombudsman.org/static_pages/ombudsman.cfm.

CHAPTER 16: THE 10 BEST QUESTIONS

to Recognize Elder Abuse

Some rob you with a gun, some with a fountain pen.
—Woody Guthrie

No one likes to think that their loved one might be subject to maltreatment under any circumstances. Unfortunately, an estimated 2 million older Americans are victims of physical, psychological, financial, and other forms of abuse and neglect. This estimate is probably low, since most experts believe there are up to five times more cases that go unreported every year. The term "elder abuse" covers these types of mistreatments: physical abuse, emotional abuse, sexual abuse, exploitation (theft, fraud, and coercion), neglect, abandonment, and self-neglect.

Elder abuse is clearly against the law. But enforcement is often difficult, especially when the victim has advanced Alzheimer's disease.

In long-term care facilities, AD residents often can't express themselves well enough to tell authorities, can't clearly remember the incidents, or can easily be discredited as "imagining it." Research has shown that older adults (over age eighty) who need more physical assistance and have significant cognitive decline are the most likely abuse victims. About 75 percent of elder abuse victims are frail, and 60 percent have dementia.

One of caregivers' greatest worries is that their loved one with advanced Alzheimer's will become a victim of abuse or neglect while she is living in a nursing home or other long-term care facility. The following Best Questions have been adapted from the National Center on Elder Abuse's list of warning signs, the com-

> **THE QUESTION DOCTOR SAYS:**
>
> If you have concerns, trust your instincts and don't be afraid to ask questions. When you report abuse or neglect to police or other authorities, be prepared for **their** questions. Have the facts ready, including the answers to the questions of who, what, when, where, and how often the abuse has occurred. Keep detailed notes as documentation of what you have observed or use your cellphone to capture photos and video images.

prehensive "Elder Assessment Instrument," and other sources credited in the Resources section beginning on page 273. Ask yourself these questions as you contemplate the possibility of abuse or neglect happening to your loved one.

Call the police or 911 immediately if you think your loved one or another nursing home resident is in immediate, life-threatening danger. If you suspect abuse or neglect, know that nursing homes are required by federal law to have intervention strategies and regular monitoring to prevent elder abuse.

There should be a responsible person at the facility whom you can talk with. If not, or if you are still unsatisfied, call local adult protective services, ask your local Agency on Aging for contacts to local law enforcement authorities, or call a long-term care ombudsman, usually available through local government agencies. The National Center on Elder Abuse's toll-free hotline is 1-800-677-1116.

〉〉〉THE 10 BEST QUESTIONS
to Recognize Elder Abuse

1. Is my loved one the victim of possible *unintentional* neglect?

Residents living in facilities where the staff is overworked and understaffed are more likely suffer from unintentional neglect. This type of neglect includes forgetting to include residents in social activities or meals, withholding attention or care, or staff members simply not being responsive fast enough to calls for assistance or complaints.

2. Is my loved one a victim of possible *intentional* neglect?

Intentional neglect includes a lack of assistance for toileting, feeding, bathing, or walking. It also includes situations where the staff purposely ignores call bells or cries for help. Intentional neglect is also the failure to provide food, water, clothing, or medications for a dependent person.

3. Could my loved one be suffering from self-neglect?

Unfortunately, some elderly people, including those with advanced Alzheimer's disease, may neglect to take care of themselves properly. If you have been your loved one's primary caregiver before her admittance into the nursing home, you already know that she forgets to take her medications, wear the right clothing, or attend to her bathing and toileting needs.

Now you've had her admitted into a long-term care facility to make sure she is actually cared for. She probably is, but be vigilant that an overworked staff is not contributing to your loved one's self-neglect.

4. Does my loved one have bedsores?

Bedsores, also called pressure sores or decubitus ulcers, are an indictor of substandard care. If left untreated, bedsores can produce craters that expose the muscles, tendons, and bones and the person can die from severe infections. Although bedsores are common in nursing homes, they are not acceptable. Bedsores can be prevented by routine hygiene and care, changing a bedridden person's position regularly, and insuring that he has adequate nutrition.

5. Are there bruises or other signs of physical abuse on my loved one?

Physical abuse is defined as a staff member or outsider intentionally harming a resident by hitting, shoving, force-feeding, scratching, slapping, or spitting. Another example is roughly handling a resident during care, medicine administration, or moving them to a different location. Bruises on the hips or arms may indicate falls caused by staff inattention or aggressive acts such as shoving. Wrists that are bruised may mean the person was physically restrained by cuffs or bedrails.

Elderly people do bruise more easily and heal more slowly than younger people, especially if they have poor circulation. But bruises should never be ignored, especially a consistent pattern of bruising.

Other signs of physical abuse are pressure marks, broken bones, cuts, and burns. None of these are acceptable under any circumstance. Each time you visit your loved one, look her over for any of these telltale signs.

6. Has my loved one suddenly withdrawn from normal activities or seem unusually depressed?

Emotional or psychological abuse involves verbally browbeating, belittling, cursing, ridiculing, or ignoring a resident. In nursing homes, this type of abuse usually involves threatening punishment or withholding food and other basic needs.

This may be a hard question to answer. You have to try to separate out these warning signs of emotional abuse from the effects of ongoing mental decline caused by the Alzheimer's disease, which includes these symptoms.

Watch carefully to see if your loved one acts very fearful of any particular person or staff member. This can be a giveaway clue that the signs you're seeing are the result of abuse, not Alzheimer's mental decline. You'll be able to judge the situation over time, especially if you see your loved one frequently.

7. Is there evidence of unreported or unapproved use of restraints on my loved one?

Nursing homes use both physical restraints and chemical/medication restraints to make residents more manageable. Because of the problem behaviors associated with late-stage Alzheimer's, your loved one may have to be restrained without your prior knowledge or approval.

Physical restraints include leg, arm, vest, and jacket restraints, waist belts, hand mitts, cuffs, wheelchair safety bars, bedrails, and lap pillows. Some negligent nursing home workers find other ways to restrict movement for "problem people," such as parking their wheelchairs in tight corners.

Chemical restraints are even a bigger danger because they are more difficult to detect and can interfere with prescribed medications. You don't want your loved one sedated for the convenience of the nursing home staff or as punishment.

A doctor's prescription is required for both chemical and physical restraints, and a restrained resident should be closely monitored. Unfortunately, the use of restraints is fairly common and can result in personal injury to frail bodies. Restraints should rarely, if ever, be used except in emergency situations.

8. Is my loved one suddenly losing weight for no apparent reason?

There are many reasons for weight loss in nursing home residents, such as serious illness, poor food, and dehydration. Alzheimer's residents also lose weight due to forgetfulness and a declining appetite.

Sudden weight loss, for whatever reason, is a serious and potentially life-threatening condition. Ensure as much as possible that the cause of weight loss is related to AD and not due to neglect or the withholding of food from your loved one. He may need more assistance with eating than he is receiving from the staff. Regardless of the cause, this condition needs immediate medical attention.

9. Is my loved one the victim of sexual abuse?

Sexual abuse is defined as the improper touching or coercion to perform sexual acts. This may be difficult even to contemplate. Telltale signs include bruises around the breasts or in the genital area or the onset of sexually transmitted diseases.

10. Are my loved one's financial assets being misappropriated or stolen?

Financial abuse is the embezzlement or stealing of a resident's money and is made more likely by not placing a resident's funds in a separate, interest-bearing account, as usually required in nursing homes. In other situations, residents' personal funds are deliberately misplaced or misused without the persons' consent or knowledge.

Look for sudden changes in financial accounts or large bank withdrawals. Other clues are altered wills and trusts and checks written as "cash," "loans," or "gifts."

Theft of residents' clothing, personal property, or jewelry is unfortunately fairly common in nursing homes. Do everything you can to keep valuables out of the nursing home altogether, especially as your loved one declines into an increasingly inattentive and forgetful state of mind.

❯ The Magic Question

Have I seen any incidences of yelling, hitting, or shouting either among staff members or against residents?

If you've witnessed recent examples of abusive or neglectful behavior by the staff toward other residents, this will help you to determine if your suspicions about your loved one are off base or on target. Listen in at the nurses' central station or other places where staff members gather to chat informally. If they sound disgruntled, argue frequently, or seem aggressive toward one another, they may also be taking their anger out on residents.

Look for signs of alcohol or drug use among staff members. Observe if staffers seem to overcontrol or isolate some residents or appear to be indifferent or hostile to residents' calls for assistance.

Your observations aren't positive proof but may confirm what your gut is telling you from the other warning signs you've seen.

CONCLUSION

Elder abuse can happen to anyone. Your loved one isn't responsible and didn't cause it.

The best thing you can do to prevent your loved one from being abused or neglected is to stay alert and not turn a blind eye to obvious warning signs. Knowing what to look for by asking yourself these Best Questions may help ease your fears of a worst-case scenario and increase the likelihood you'll take action if neglect or abuse does occur.

Patricia Callone, long-time caregiver and co-author of Alzheimer's Disease, the Dignity Within: *A Handbook for Caregivers, Family, and Friends*, concludes, "Elder abuse is hidden most of the time because no one likes to talk about it."

IT'S ALL IN THE FAMILY, TOO

Family members and caregivers, most often adult children or spouses, are statistically the most frequent abusers of their vulnerable elderly relatives. Primary caregivers are under tremendous pressure and can suffer from extreme stress, frustration, and depression, which they take out on their loved ones.

Sometimes family members just simply go bad, too. Caregiver Elaine Marshall of Leesburg, Virginia, recalls what happened after her mother's Alzheimer's diagnosis. "My sister was able to take 80 percent of our mother's liquid assets without Mom's knowledge. For example, once my sister charged seventy-five hundred dollars in cash advances for her personal use and charged about a thousand dollars more in local stores. We thought we could trust my sister and never dreamed this would happen."

THE 10 BEST RESOURCES

Administration on Aging. "Elder Abuse." www.aoa.gov/eldfam/Elder_ Rights/Elder_Abuse/Elder_Abuse.asp.

Brandl, Bonnie, et al. *Elder Abuse Detection and Intervention: A Collaborative Approach*. New York: Springer, 2007.

Johnson, Kelly Dedel. "Financial Crimes Against the Elderly." U.S. Department of Justice, Office of Community Oriented Policing Services. www.cops.usdoj.gov/pdf/pop/e07042443.pdf.

National Center on Elder Abuse. "15 Questions and Answers About Elder Abuse." www.ncea.aoa.gov/NCEAroot/Main_Site/pdf/publication/FINAL %206-06-05%203-18-0512-10-04qa.pdf.

National Center on Elder Abuse. "Elder Abuse Awareness Kit: A Resource Kit for Protecting Older People and People with Disabilities." www.ncea .aoa.gov/NCEAroot/Main_Site/pdf/basics/speakers.pdf.

National Center on Elder Abuse. "Factsheets and Publications." www .ncea.aoa.gov/NCEAroot/Main_Site/Find_Help/Resources/Factsheets_Pub lications.aspx.

National Center on Elder Abuse. "State Resource Directory on Elder Abuse Prevention." www.ncea.aoa.gov/NCEAroot/Main_Site/Find_Help/State_Resources.aspx.

National Citizens' Coalition for Nursing Home Reform. "Abuse and Neglect." www.nccnhr.org/public/50_156_450.cfm.

National Institute on Aging, "Abuse Associated with Increased Risk of Death for Older People." http://www.nia.nih.gov/NewsAndEvents/PressReleases/PR19980804Abuse.htm.

Wiehe, Vernon R. "Elder Abuse." In *Understanding Family Violence: Treating and Preventing Partner, Child, Sibling, and Elder Abuse.* Thousand Oaks, Calif.: Sage Publications, 1998.

PART IV:

Caring for the Caregiver

The national statistics on the numbers of caregivers in the United States are staggering. According to the Family Caregiver Alliance, there are an estimated total of 52 million informal, unpaid caregivers in the United States alone.

Of these, nearly 9 million caregivers are tending to the needs of family members and friends with Alzheimer's disease or other dementias. Six to seven million unpaid family caregivers tend to the advanced needs of people who need assistance with bathing, toileting, and eating. An estimated 59 to 75 percent of all caregivers are women.

Experts predict that unpaid caregiving will continue as the largest source of long-term care services in the United States, with an estimated increase of 85 percent between 2000 and 2050 as the aging baby boom generation becomes increasingly memory challenged and frail.

These statistics are interesting but not especially useful if you are a primary caregiver. It's another Monday morning, and your loved one has made yet another mess that you now have to clean up. That's the reality of caregiving, a usually thankless job with no time clock that lets you punch out at the end of the day.

If this sounds familiar, this section and lists of Best Questions are for you. Chapter 17 discusses the questions to ask yourself to assess your emotional health and stress, which many caregivers overlook or ignore until their own health has been damaged.

The next chapter explains the Best Questions to share with your partner when one spouse has AD. There's also a separate list of Best

Questions about sex and intimacy to help you start a dialogue on these sensitive issues.

Chapter 19 will help you to assess your aging parents' situations from afar if you are a long-distance caregiver. Many adult children don't know when to react or what to look for as they try to determine how much care their overly proud, silent, or resistant parents actually need.

Many people touched by AD contemplate joining a support group. Chapter 20 will guide you in your choices.

The Question Doctor sincerely hopes the Best Questions in this section will give you personal strength, comfort, and knowledge as you travel down the often-difficult road of caregiving.

CHAPTER 17: THE 10 BEST QUESTIONS

for a Caregiver's Emotional Health

> Reality is the leading cause of stress amongst those in
> touch with it.
>
> —Lily Tomlin

Caregivers react to the initial diagnosis of Alzheimer's disease and deal with later problem behaviors in many different ways. Chances are your emotional roller-coaster ride has included feelings of sadness, anger, frustration, helplessness, despair, and perhaps depression. Jacqueline Marcell, the author of *Elder Rage* and a long-time caregiver, says, "The importance of care for the caregiver is huge because of all the stress you are under."

Seventy percent of those with AD live at home, so the impact of this illness extends to millions of family members, friends, and caregivers. Studies consistently show higher levels of depression and other mental health problems among caregivers than for others not providing care to loved ones. Depression is the most common psychological disorder, with up to 40 percent of dementia caregivers reportedly suffering from emotional stress and depression.

You may feel strong and capable, yet still be burdened by non-stop demands for your caregiving. Not only do you have to deal with your loved one's changing emotions, personality transformation, and late-stage mood swings, but you must also protect your own emotional health.

One factor that affects your emotional reactions to caregiving is how close you felt to the person with AD before she got sick. For example, if there are unresolved issues with your mother, they are bound to affect you now as you contemplate the enormity of caring for her over a long time and at great personal sacrifice.

Another consideration that affects your emotions is whether or not you volunteered for this job. You may feel resentful because you were recruited or felt pressured by a parent or older brother or sister. The needs of other dependents, such as your own children or spouse, add to your stress. And lastly, think about how much outside support you get and need, such as strong family ties or belonging to a good AD support group. Many caregivers get little or no financial support for their thousands of hours of devoted labor.

If this sounds familiar, ask yourself the following Best Questions. They will help you to better understand your own emotional state, as well as make a better-informed decision about whether or not you need outside or professional help for your own chronic stress or depression.

〉〉〉THE 10 BEST QUESTIONS
for a Caregiver's Emotional Health

1. What was my emotional state before my loved one's diagnosis of Alzheimer's disease?

One way to get your sense of balance back is to reflect on who you were and what your emotional state was before this diagnosis. Maybe you were overstressed in a dead-end job, arguing constantly with your defiant teenager, or barely hanging on to a rocky marriage. Or perhaps life was good, full of grandchildren, church activities, and postretirement travel.

Think of this question as an emotional audit that will let you put your past emotional stability and the ups and downs of your prior relationship with your loved one into the proper perspective. This reality check will keep you from romanticizing or mourning your past as the "good old days"—which may not have been quite as great as you remember.

This honest self-reflection is your starting point—square one—for the following Best Questions.

2. What coping strategies have been most successful for me in the past?

What were your greatest emotional and personal challenges before your loved one's AD diagnosis? How did you handle those challenges? What did you do especially well and feel proud about?

Start from a position of personal strength based on your most positive past experiences. Then you'll feel more solid as you face up to the current situation of caring for your loved one despite her increasingly difficult behaviors and memory lapses. Analyze your past successes so you can use these same coping strategies again.

3. How do I feel about my loved one's mental and physical changes?

You aren't required to like the changes you may see happening in your loved one. Over time, the personality of most AD patients is transformed from the person you once knew and loved into a demanding, vile-tempered stranger.

But instead of focusing on your loved one's emotions and changes, think for once about your own feelings. Try to sort them out, either through quiet self-reflection, discussion in a support group, or talking with another family member, friend, or professional counselor.

4. How well am I handling other people's reactions to my loved one's Alzheimer's disease?

How the people closest to you react to your loved one's AD will affect your emotional well-being. Family members and friends can be great sources of support but can also cause you additional emotional hardship.

For example, your brother may freak out about your mother's

Alzheimer's, but all he talks about is his own genetic risks for AD instead of offering empathy for you cleaning up more of your mother's messes today. You may be embarrassed by your mother's strange behavior in public places. Friends may pull away from her as if she were contagious or only talk baby talk to her. Others act like nothing's wrong, fearful of discussing the often taboo topic of mental illness.

Reflecting on this question may help you realize another source of stress you may have been overlooking.

5. Where can I get help? Who are my best resources for support?

Talk to your family doctor, AD specialist, support group, family and friends, or a trusted religious leader about getting help. Don't be afraid to ask for help or actively seek it out.

You deserve support as much as your loved one does. If you don't take care of yourself, it will mean that both of you will suffer.

6. What am I denying or avoiding about this diagnosis? (Stage 1)

After a diagnosis of Alzheimer's disease, the abstractness of death becomes more real. No one likes to face her own death or contemplate the death of her beloved parent or spouse. Psychologists tell us that it's human nature to deal with this harsh reality first by going into shock or extreme surprise, and then by denial, pretending this isn't really happening.

What matters most is how well you cope with first your loved one's AD diagnosis and second with the possibly frightening prospects of full-time, long-term caregiving.

Getting over your own denial will help you move to the next stages and ultimately find peace of mind. At the same time, realize that one characteristic behavior of AD is denial that there's anything wrong. It may be especially difficult for your loved one to move beyond this stage.

THE QUESTION DOCTOR SAYS:

In psychiatrist Dr. Elisabeth Kübler-Ross's groundbreaking 1969 book *On Death and Dying,* she outlined her five stages of grief as the pattern most people experience as they face a life-threatening illness or deal with grief.

The five stages applied to caregiving emotions are:

1. **Shock and denial.** The initial stage: "This can't be happening to us/me."
2. **Anger.** "Why me? This isn't fair. I want my own life, too."
3. **Bargaining.** "Just let me live through another day."
4. **Depression.** "Why even bother anymore?"
5. **Acceptance.** "I'm going to be OK and live through this."

Not everyone moves neatly through the stages in an orderly fashion or at the same pace. For example, you might experience anger (stage 2) and then depression (stage 4), go backward to denial (stage 1), or get stuck at bargaining (stage 3).

Best Questions 6 through 10 use Dr. Kübler-Ross's stages to help you get in touch with your deepest emotional responses to caregiving stress. As President Ronald Reagan's wife, Nancy, once said about her husband's Alzheimer's disease, it's "the long good-bye." This gradual decline of your loved one puts you through a slow-motion grieving process as the person you knew slips away. As the caregiver, be aware that your loved one is also going through these same stages, too.

7. How can I channel my anger into a more positive experience for both of us? (Stage 2)

Nearly everyone goes through this stage. As the caregiver, you may be angry at your loved one, at yourself, at other family members, at your doctors, or at God for letting Alzheimer's happen to good people. It may seem that God is unjustly punishing you and your loved one, especially if you believe you've faithfully followed your religious observances or lived by the Golden Rule.

Try to channel your anger into positive actions, like researching

Alzheimer's disease, eating better, reading books with your loved one, starting a private journal of your thoughts and feelings, talking with others, or assembling a family photo album.

It's very important to move beyond this stage. The people who get stuck here are the most likely to experience severe depression, feel helpless, or abuse their loved ones. Get professional help if you feel your anger is out of control.

Alzheimer's disease itself is characterized by angry outbursts and sometimes violent behaviors toward others. As the caregiver, it's tough not to be angry in return.

8. What am I bargaining for, either consciously or unconsciously? (Stage 3)

Dr. Kübler-Ross describes this stage in *On Death and Dying:*

> The bargaining is really an attempt to postpone; it has to include a prize offered "for good behavior," it also sets a self-imposed deadline . . . like children who say, "I will never fight with my sister again". . . . Most bargains are made with God and usually kept a secret.

As a caregiver, your mental script for unconscious bargaining may run something like this: "If I take good care of my father, it will delay his dementia." Fear is a powerful force at work here, including fears of the unknown, worsening AD symptoms, putting your loved one in a nursing home, the fear of death, and personal fears about your own future.

Bargaining is another potentially dangerous place to get stuck. It can lead to an endless loop of trying to do the "right things" or going the extra mile when you can't actually control the disease's progression or your loved one's reactions to it.

9. How can I better cope with my feelings of being overly stressed and depressed? (Stage 4)

You may be so concerned about caring for your loved one's needs that you lose sight of your own well-being. At-home caregiver Elaine Marshall of Leesburg, Virginia, says, "I get depressed and cry sometimes just looking at my mom. She's so helpless, vulnerable, and totally dependent on me, not at all the person I grew up with." Long-distance caregiver Jim Winter of Perth, Western Australia, agrees. He says, "I usually end up just wanting to cry. It's absolutely terrible."

Over time, these emotions can lead to serious stress and depression. The American Medical Association says that caregiver stress is characterized by frequently feeling lonely, overwhelmed, irritable, sad, empty, or tired. You may also have little or no pleasure in life, crying spells, worries about leaving your loved one alone, and feeling worthless or suicidal. Physical symptoms include shortness of breath, appetite changes, and feeling weak.

Dr. Richard Stoltz, the director for military and family health at the National Naval Medical Center in Bethesda, Maryland, comments, "The failure to acknowledge the potential difficulties of adjusting to changes can contribute to a person becoming overwhelmed."

Seek professional help if your stress or depression is interfering with your life. The Family Caregiver Alliance cites studies that have shown that counseling and support groups in combination with respite and other services can help caregivers remain in their caregiving roles longer and with less stress and more satisfaction.

10. What steps can I take to accept my loved one's Alzheimer's disease? How can I put to rest any feelings of guilt? (Stage 5)

Dr. Kübler-Ross believed that it's the acknowledgment of grief about change or a pending loss that holds the key to acceptance with dignity and grace.

Another version of this Best Question is, "How can I treat myself with more compassion?" Many caregivers are stricken by guilt, regardless of how effective or dedicated their caregiving is. Deep inside you may have unconsciously placed yourself in the impossible role of being personally responsible for your loved one's life and death. Your grief is only compounded by this unwarranted guilt. In turn, your guilt drains your energy to work through your emotions and support your loved one.

Mark Gorkin—Maryland author, licensed clinical social worker, and self-proclaimed Stress Doc—says, "Caregivers frequently cycle between anger, due to the unreasonable demands of caregiving, and being in a state of chronic guilt and stress for not being able to do it all."

› The Magic Question

How can I feel my best today?

Many caregivers allow their loved one's disease and symptoms to determine how they feel.

You can take back control of your emotions with this question. It puts you in the driver's seat and makes you an active player rather than a passive victim of Alzheimer's disease.

Start each day with this Magic Question to find your own emotional well-being, self-acceptance, and a sense of inner peace.

CONCLUSION

Caregiving is a very stressful experience for most people. Yet studies also show the beneficial effects include feeling positive about helping a disabled loved one, feeling appreciated by other family members or friends, and reaching a new understanding of the person in your life who has Alzheimer's disease.

Your loved one's diagnosis of Alzheimer's disease can be emotionally transformative for you as the caregiver. You may rise to this challenge as you never expected you could and find new, meaningful ways of connecting, even in the last stages of Alzheimer's disease.

Author and Alzheimer specialist Dr. Peter Whitehouse concludes, "You, the caregiver, can find yourself as a human being in new and different ways."

THE 10 BEST RESOURCES

Alzheimer's Disease Education and Referral Center. "Caregiver Guide." www.nia.nih.gov/Alzheimers/Publications/caregiverguide.htm.

American Geriatrics Society. "The Alzheimer's Disease Caregiver." www.americangeriatrics.org/education/forum/alzcare.shtml.

American Medical Association. "Caregiver Self-Assessment Questionnaire: How Are You?" www.ama-assn.org/ama1/pub/upload/mm/433/caregiver_english.pdf.

Family Caregiver Alliance. "Caregiver's Guide to Understanding Dementia Behaviors." www.caregiver.org/caregiver/jsp/content_node.jsp?nodeid=391.

Family Caregiver Alliance. "Caregiving and Depression." www.caregiver.org/caregiver/jsp/content_node.jsp?nodeid=393.

Kübler-Ross, Elisabeth. *On Death and Dying.* New York: Scribner, 1997.

Mace, Nancy, and Peter Rabins. "How Caring for an Impaired Person Affects You." In *The 36-Hour Day: A Family Guide To Caring for Persons with Alzheimer Disease, Related Dementing Illnesses, and Memory Loss in Later Life,* 4th ed. Baltimore, Md.: The Johns Hopkins University Press, 2006.

MetLife. "Alzheimer's Disease: Caregiving Challenges." www.metlife.com/FileAssets/MMI/MMISYCAlzheimerCareChallenges07.pdf.

Morris, Virginia, and Robert M. Butler. "Caring for the Caregiver." In *How to Care for Aging Parents.* New York: Workman Publishing, 2004.

Oliver, Rose, and Frances A. Bock. *Coping with Alzheimer's: A Caregiver's Emotional Survival Guide.* Chatsworth, Calif.: Wilshire Book Company, 1989.

CHAPTER 18: THE 10 BEST QUESTIONS

When One Spouse Has
Alzheimer's Disease

To know another is not to know that person's face, but to know that person's heart.

—Chinese proverb

Alzheimer's disease often has not just one victim, the person with AD, but two—the spouse or long-term partner. The devastating impact that Alzheimer's has on even the most iron-clad relationships is rarely discussed or acknowledged, but it happens. The private pain the spouse of an AD patient feels often goes unexpressed and underappreciated.

The lack of a healthy outlet or a chance to talk about this strain after a diagnosis of early stage AD or MCI adds tremendously to the stresses felt later by the well spouse, who may spend years as the full-time primary caregiver. The caregiver's resentments are likely to be more profound because the "good glue" of a heartfelt dialogue never happened.

In other words, now—while you, the person with AD, or you, the spouse, are still basically OK—this is your window of opportunity to communicate. Medical experts say you probably still have time—maybe one year, maybe five years—to communicate and go about your daily lives with minimal assistance.

Ask each other the following Best Questions. These questions work equally well for both people to ask each other in a two-way conversation. The assumption here is that the AD is still mild enough to make this dialogue possible.

THE QUESTION DOCTOR SAYS:

Take this conversation slowly or just one question at a time. You might also select a single Best Question that really resonates with you and skip the rest.

The most important thing is that you are having this conversation at all. Consider video-taping or recording yourselves as a way for the caregiver to preserve memories of your good times together as a couple.

〉〉〉 THE 10 BEST QUESTIONS
When One Spouse Has Alzheimer's Disease

1. **When were we most successful in communicating with each other in the past? How can we use the same methods now to deal with this illness together?**

Reflecting on your past successes and analyzing why those communications were good ones is a positive way to start this conversation. It's common sense to build from a position of strength and hope as you seek to reestablish your connections for the future's challenges.

2. **What areas of our lives must we maintain to ensure our normalcy for as long as possible?**

Favorite routines, like going to church on Sunday, Friday night visits with the grandkids, or "meatloaf Mondays" can become precious when they are potentially threatened.

Few couples facing Alzheimer's disease consciously consider their normal patterns and daily routines. Solve this problem together as a team by identifying your most essential core.

A MESSAGE FROM MARS AND VENUS

The biggest problem between men and women is this: She gives an answer and he assumes there's a period and that's the end of the point. That's never the end of the point, she's just warming up.

—DR. JOHN GRAY, RELATIONSHIP GURU AND AUTHOR OF THE BESTSELLING BOOK
   MEN ARE FROM MARS, WOMEN ARE FROM VENUS

3. What changes in our relationship do we need to discuss, understand, and accept?

Your past roles and the division of labor in your partnership may be turned upside down after a diagnosis of Alzheimer's. You can't change or control this disease, but you can at least consider how to cope with it together.

4. What is this like for you?

This question can uncover a hornet's nest of complaints, feelings, or a silent shrug. As the spouse, it may not have occurred to you to ask a question so direct and simple. If you have AD, you may be so self-absorbed and frightened that you haven't adequately considered your spouse's perspective.

Relationship advisors Dr. Scott Peck and Shannon Peck of San Diego, California, commented, "There are many ways to bring the empowering combination of kindness and love into your marriage. One way is to ask simple direct questions . . . this can bring great healing power."

5. How can we help each other deal with the additional stress in our lives?

It's human nature to take the additional stress and fear of the unknown out on each other. Back up and analyze if this is happening in your relationship. If so, how can you get reunited as a team facing this diagnosis together instead of two lonely and isolated people, both angry and afraid?

6. How can I show you that I love you?

Be a "love pharmacist" and dispense your hugs like good medicine. If you want more, see the 10 Best Questions in this chapter on sex and intimacy, page 194.

7. How can we still enjoy being together and have fun?

What's something silly or easy that the two of you can do just like the old days? Get your favorite takeout pizza, rent your favorite movie, and watch it together without once thinking, "Alzheimer's." Now do it again.

8. What can I do to help you now and later?

Just knowing that the loved one's AD temper tantrums aren't personal can greatly relieve some spouses who might think they somehow are responsible. Finding ways to overcome your own anxiety attacks and letting the storms pass will help both the person with AD and the spouse/caregiver tremendously. This question also works as a springboard for financial and legal discussions.

9. Do we need professional counseling or other help for our marriage?

If you are already seeing an AD specialist, such as a geriatric psychiatrist, take advantage of her expertise and book an appointment just to discuss your marital difficulties. As the AD patient, this frank discussion will help you understand how your behavior changes are likely to affect your spouse. As the spouse/caregiver, you need practical advice for coping with current and future difficulties.

10. What old rules do we need to break? What new rules do we need to establish?

Over time, nonverbal communication becomes increasingly important as people with AD start to lose their language capabilities. Your reliance on words and abstract meanings in your communication won't work as well any longer.

Old rules to break might include this reliance on words for communication. New rules include finding a different way of communicating that relies on simplified yes/no questions and a prearranged set of nonverbal hand signals or gestures. As the AD worsens, these new rules won't be foolproof either. Discuss your own old and new rules—the ones that work for you.

❯ The Magic Question

What are you afraid to ask me? What are we not talking about that needs to be addressed?

Most couples fear the verbal and physical rage that often accompanies AD. The loss of reasoning and judgment capabilities is also frightening, as well as the prospect of the money woes caused by upcoming long-term care costs.

These are very real fears, and talking about them won't make them go away. But this conversation can help you plan together in advance as much as possible while you are still a team.

THE 10 BEST QUESTIONS FOR SEXUAL HEALTH AND INTIMACY AFTER ALZHEIMER'S

Changing sexual relations and lost intimacy in a relationship touched by Alzheimer's disease is one of the most underdiscussed challenges that caregivers experience. Many couples struggle to maintain normalcy, including their sexual relationship, after a diagnosis of early stage AD. But they often face difficult obstacles, including loss of desire, stress, depression, and a breakdown in communications.

As Dr. Julia Heiman, executive director of the Kinsey Institute for Research in Sex, Gender, and Reproduction, says, "The value of asking questions for couples in intimate relationships is that it's a way of trying to see the other person as they are . . . No matter how long they've been together, that's really crucial."

Asking each other the following Best Questions can help you to rebuild communication channels while you resume or continue intimate relations with your loved one. Keep in mind that most early stage AD patients can expect some time of nearly symptom-free living. Why not spend some of that time exchanging hugs and kisses?

1. **How can we best communicate with each other about our needs for sex and intimacy?**
    Women tend to romanticize about sex while men have a body-centered or recreational approach. These natural differences between men and women explain why talking about sex can be tricky.

    Your best communications might be using no words at all. Simple nonverbal cues, such as a "come hither" glance or wink, help to smooth misunderstandings and clarify your amorous intentions.

2. **Are you comfortable being intimate again?**
    If you are no longer having regular sexual relations or have stopped touching, this question will help you to find out why.

3. **How can we redefine and restart our intimacy and sexual pleasure again?**
    If the answer to question 2 was yes, now it's time to do something about it. To get in the mood, try the following:

    > Enjoy a romantic candlelight dinner

    > Offer a long sensual massage

> Watch an erotic video together

> Try new sexual positions

> Book a romantic vacation or a quick get-away trip

4. **What physical changes in your body do you want me to know about?**
   Older bodies may mean sore knees, less natural lubrication for women, or diminished stamina for men. This is a gentle way to approach a tough topic.

5. **What can I do to please you?**
   If you focus on mutual pleasure, sex becomes fun again. Intimacy is proven good medicine—for both of you.

   Harriette Cole, author of the nationally syndicated advice column *Sense and Sensitivity* and the creative director of *Ebony* magazine, agrees. She says, "I think questions are very important in all relationships, especially in intimate relationships."

6. **What's the craziest or funniest thing we could do to show our love for each other?**
   Rediscover your passion by having fun together. Put aside your worries and fears so you can live in this moment of passion together—again.

7. **Is there anything off-limits now that was okay before?**
   If you don't ask each other this question, your unspoken assumptions about what's acceptable and what's not can cause misunderstandings. Talk this question out without criticism or bringing up your past sexual or marital problems.

8. **We agree we both have a low interest in sex right now. What can we do to get back on track?**
   This Best Question applies to the times that neither of you wants sexual relations. Assuming you want to try again, this question clears the air while keeping the door open for later.

9. **We can't agree about having sexual relations or being intimate. How can we work it out?**
   Even if you've lost sexual desire, you can still be intimate and show affection through kissing, touching, stroking, cuddling, hugging, and massaging each other, or by sharing loving words of comfort and hope.

(continued)

10. Do we need professional help?
Consider the option of talking with a geriatric psychiatrist, a professional therapist, or marriage counselor. Unresolved sexual tensions can result in emotional strain and distance in long-term relationships.

The Magic Question
What sexual fears are we not talking about that need to be addressed?
Not talking about sexual problems puts a tremendous strain on your relationship, just at the very time when you need closeness, good communication, and each other more than ever.

CONCLUSION

Coping with Alzheimer's disease is heartbreaking. This unwanted and uninvited houseguest has invaded your lives and your relationship. The person with AD becomes a stranger, not the person you were or the person you loved and married. Perhaps the person with AD is already displaying irrational behavior or sudden rages.

While you still can, cherish this time together. Focus on your loving relationship to help you deal with the darker days ahead.

THE 10 BEST RESOURCES

Alzheimer Spouse. "Message Boards." www.thealzheimerspouse.com/vanilla forum.

Alzheimer's Association, "Changes in Relationships." www.alz.org/living_with_alzheimers_changes_in_relationships.asp.

Alzheimer's Association. "Families and Friends." See the section "Your Partner." www.alz.org/living_with_alzheimers_families_and_friends.asp.

Alzheimer's Association. "Sexuality and Intimacy Issues in Alzheimer's Disease." Resource list. www.alz.org/national/documents/SexandIntimac_RL.doc.

Cohen, Donna, and Carl Eisdorfer. *The Loss of Self: A Family Resource for the Care of Alzheimer's Disease and Related Disorders.* New York: W. W. Norton, 2002.

Davidson, Ann. *A Curious Kind of Widow: Loving a Man with Advanced Alzheimer's.* McKinleyville, Calif.: Fithian Press, 2006.

Gray, John. *Men Are from Mars, Women Are from Venus: The Classic Guide to Understanding the Opposite Sex.* New York: Harper Paperbacks, 2004.

Mayo Clinic. "Intimacy Important for All." www.mayoclinic.com/health/alzheimers/AZ00061.

Wallace, Meredith. "Sexuality Assessment for Older Adults." *Try This.* Issue 10, revised 2007. Hartford Institute for Geriatric Nursing. www.hartfordign.org/publications/trythis/issue10.pdf.

Well Spouse Foundation. "Support Programs." www.wellspouse.org/index.php?option=com_content&task=section&id=8&Itemid=37.

CHAPTER 19: THE 10 BEST QUESTIONS
for Long-Distance Caregivers—
Does Dad Need Help?

I have a photographic memory, but once in a while I
forget to take off the lens cap.

—Milton Berle

According to the Family Caregiver Alliance, between 5 and 7 million people in the United States are long-distance caregivers. Long-distance caregiving is defined as living more than one hour from an aging parent who needs assistance. This phenomenon is growing as families increasingly scatter across the country.

If you are one of these long-distance caregivers, you probably worry about your father or mother and wonder if he or she is telling you everything you need to know. If your parent has just received a diagnosis of early stage AD or mild cognitive impairment (MCI), your worry scale has probably been ratcheted up a few notches, too. You dread the call in the middle of the night about Mom's kitchen fire or Dad's broken hip.

Linda Dano, daytime television's star of *One Life to Live, As the World Turns, All My Children,* and *General Hospital,* recalls her experiences with her father's Alzheimer's disease more than ten years ago. "My mother, like all mothers and fathers—I think they must go to this class on how to never tell your children anything because they don't want to worry you—she didn't tell me what was going on. I lived in New York and they lived in California. She wasn't telling me that he was banging cupboards in the middle of the night and threatening her. It was like something out of a Stephen King novel."

Ms. Dano's experience is all too common. As a long-distance caregiver, you may have to coordinate care and community services for your parent by phone, as well as provide his emotional and spiritual support. Talking and listening are some of the most important things you can do.

Telepathy doesn't help much for long-distance caregivers, but the following Best Questions will. These questions will help you to understand from afar what's really going on—even when you can't be there.

Knowing what to ask when you talk to your parents on the telephone will ease your own stress and guilt and help you to make well-informed decisions about what to do next. These questions should not replace medical guidance or professional counseling services.

It's also important to note that the following questions assume that the person you are talking with does not have significantly impaired cognitive functioning or damaged reasoning capabilities. Adjust these questions as needed and add your own questions to fit your circumstances, your parent's personality, and your relationship with him.

〉〉〉 THE 10 BEST QUESTIONS
for Long-Distance Caregivers—Does Dad Need Help?

1. How are you feeling? What's the latest with your health condition?
Perhaps your dad has long-standing vision problems, is recovering from a stroke, or has high blood pressure. It's easier to start a question about an established physical condition than launch into an investigation of his deteriorating mental condition.

Getting him to open up now will increase the likelihood that he'll be less evasive on tougher questions later. Just don't get sidetracked by discussing only his physical ailments, which some seniors like to do.

THE QUESTION DOCTOR SAYS:

Your loved ones may still be reluctant to tell you what's going on. This is especially true if they have been delaying going to the doctor for a formal diagnosis. Your well parent may not understand the behavioral symptoms of Alzheimer's and be afraid that your dad has just flipped out.

If you suspect this is the case, try a few additional introductory questions the next time you talk, such as, "When's the last time Dad went to the doctor?" or "Has Mom changed recently and you aren't telling me about it?" or "Does Dad seem more forgetful lately?" and "Are you going to see the doctor soon?"

Gentle yet direct questions can help ease a difficult conversation if your parents are resistant or tend to gloss over problems. Use your usual small talk questions, too.

---

2. When's the last time you saw the doctor? Do you ever forget or get mixed up about your appointments?

You want to make sure he's getting good regular medical attention and at the same time hasn't progressed so far that getting to the doctor's office has become problematic. Ask someone close to your father if he's truly keeping his doctor appointments.

3. Are you taking your medications every day? Do you ever forget to take your pills (eye drops, etc.)?

Ask this important question without a condescending tone in your voice. Otherwise, your father may resent the obvious role reversal here (adult child caring for parent) or think you're being nosy.

Try gentle follow-up questions like, "If you forget, what do you do about it?" However, your father may lie and you may not know it. If you suspect this problem, seek corroboration from another person so you can be assured that your father is actually taking his prescriptions correctly and not mixing them up.

If your father is in a long-term care facility, ask the nursing supervisor if his medications need adjustment and when the doctor last reviewed your father's drugs and dosages.

4. Are you still able to get around well? Are you still driving OK? What kind of things have you been doing lately?

Listen for clues about your father's physical mobility. For example, if he tells you he's been reading or doing crossword puzzles, that's a less strenuous activity than gardening or swimming.

If he's a reader, that doesn't automatically make him more immobile, but a smart follow-up question from you based on the activities he's enjoyed in the past will give you further information on how well he's able to function independently.

Be alert to any indications of falls or injuries. If you think this is a concern, ask your father directly if he's hurt himself lately by accident.

Driving is an important separate issue for people with MCI or early stage AD. See chapter 22 for the Best Questions about driving.

5. Who's the last person you saw (besides anyone your parent lives with)? What did you do together? When was that? Did you enjoy it?

Social isolation and depression are two of the biggest problems for seniors, especially for people who live alone. If you can ask these questions with a light tone rather than sounding like an inquisitor, your father is more likely to tell you about his bridge club, church meeting, or trip to the barber.

Listen between the words for his sense of enjoyment, his ease of doing these things, if he's still driving, and how frequently he has social contacts. If your father lives in a long-term care facility, you want to know how well he's interacting with the other residents.

6. Are you sleeping well? How many hours of sleep do you get on the average per night?

Changes in sleeping habits may be an indicator of physical or mental deterioration. At minimum, not getting enough sleep is not healthy.

7. How's your appetite? What's in your refrigerator right now?

Appetite changes are another warning sign of major changes in your father's condition. By asking what's in his refrigerator, you'll have a better idea of how much meal preparation he's doing, how well he's eating, and if food is rotting because of neglect or poor appetite.

Be sure to ask about excessive weight loss or gain if this question makes sense in your father's case. Losing a lot of weight is an especially important warning sign of malnutrition or other physical changes. It is also a common side effect of the AD drugs called "cholinesterase inhibitors" (Aricept, etc.). See chapter 6.

8. Did you get your income taxes completed and mailed off? Did you get the tax assessment on your house yet? Are you having any problems with finances or making payments?

This is a tricky question about personal finances and money management. It's tricky because you don't want to pry or you may feel shy about asking, but you really need to know if your father is in financial pain or behind in his routine monthly bills.

Try connecting this question to a specific current issue or event, like paying income or property taxes, as a way to lead you into a deeper conversation about his actual financial situation. Ask someone with access to his home if he is opening his mail every day.

If your father is in financial trouble or is facing major expenses due to long-term care or medical costs, be more direct. You may need to discuss this one in person or during a family meeting. See more guidance on finances in chapter 23.

Also keep in mind that your father's mental state may be worsening. As author Daniel Kuhn of the Alzheimer's Association warns, "What is maddening to caregivers especially in the early stages is the inconsistency with respect to memory, language, and other thinking skills that we all tend to take for granted."

9. How's the house holding up? Have you made any repairs? Are you cleaning it yourself or have you hired a maid service for help?

Keeping up a household and a home are key indicators of the ability to live independently. If the house is sliding into a state of disrepair according to neighbors or other family members, this may be a warning sign of your father's declining health and his ability to continue living there.

Peeling paint doesn't automatically mean he's ready for admission to a nursing home, but this is one more clue into how well your dad is actually doing in his current situation.

10. What can I do for you, Dad? What do you need?

Your father may be the type who automatically answers, "Nothing." If that's the case, you might ask him more specific questions so he'll share what's on his mind. For example, ask about car or house repairs, taking care of the dog, or getting a different medication with fewer side effects.

Ending your phone calls with the question, "Do you know how much I love you?" sure doesn't hurt either.

❯ The Magic Question

Who is the special person I can count on to look after you?

Many long-distance caregivers believe it's vital to create a support network of people who live near your dad who he (or you) can call day or night. This network should operate for both just routine checking in and during a crisis.

Religious and volunteer organizations offer services for the elderly, as well as adult day care, some cleaning services, and home-delivered meal services. Other potential resources are social workers, social service agencies, and Area Agencies for Aging. Call Eldercare Locator at 800-677-1116 (www.eldercare.gov). Get a copy of the local telephone book in your father's area (or visit www.whitepages .com) so you'll have quick access to resources and emergency numbers where he lives.

But ultimately as a long-distance caregiver you want to know there's at least one special person who will look after your father in your absence. This special person may be his well spouse, your sister or brother who lives nearby, or a close family friend.

If you don't have a clear candidate among family members or friends, seriously consider hiring a geriatric care manager, skilled nurse, or live-in companion who will be your responsible surrogate caregiver. Be sure to stay in touch with your father's doctor on a regular basis, too.

Geriatric care managers are specialists who assess, monitor, and care for the elderly. Contact the National Association of Professional Geriatric Care Managers at 520-881-8008 (or visit www.care manager.org).

This strategy also works well if your parent is already in a long-term care facility. As experienced geriatric nurse Clare Absher observes about AD patients in nursing homes, "One key factor once

THE 10 BEST QUESTIONS WHEN YOU VISIT DAD

During your visits with your dad, keep your eyes open and ask *yourself* these questions, which have been adapted from the Alzheimer's Association's checklist:

1. Does Dad have food in the refrigerator? Is it spoiled?
2. Is he eating regular meals with a good appetite?
3. What condition is the interior and exterior of his home in?
4. Have home repairs been neglected?
5. Is he paying his bills?
6. Are there piles of unopened mail or unread newspapers?
7. Does he have regular visitors or social outings?
8. Has Dad's personal appearance changed? Does he have skin sores, burns, or seem weak?
9. Is he regularly bathing and grooming himself? Does he look unkempt, have body odor, or wear dirty clothes?
10. Is Dad still a safe driver? (See chapter 22.)

The Magic Question

Are family members or friends living near my father telling me they are worried about him?

Don't ignore their concerns. Ask these persons to describe in detail what exactly happened and when so you can understand the situation more fully and its potential seriousness.

you've put your loved one in a facility is that there's someone who stays involved. That person is your 'squeaky wheel' all the way through it and who knows all the other caregivers on a first name basis. That's really critical."

CONCLUSION

Long-distance caregivers must often rely on the telephone or e-mail as their communication link, but this can limit your ability to assess your parent's needs. Aside from true medical emergencies, you are faced with judging whether situations can be dealt with over the phone or require an in-person visit. This becomes more difficult to manage as your parent's Alzheimer's disease worsens.

The concern and love for a parent far away is often painful. Jim Winter, the director of a safety training company based in Perth, Western Australia, should know. His mother with moderate-stage Alzheimer's lives 11,349 miles and thirty-four plane-hours away in Atlanta. Jim says, "I sit here and worry about her care. But I realize that I can't be there and still have my own life. That just tears me up. I'm a problem solver, but in this case I can't. All I can do is to give suggestions to others."

Jim shares his advice for other long-distance caregivers. "Get ready for the pain. Join a local support group and get some empathy. You can also join the local Alzheimer's Association near you. Try to totally understand this disease and its progression."

And keep asking questions.

THE 10 BEST RESOURCES

AARP. "How to Deal with Long-Distance Issues." http://assets.aarp.org/external_sites/caregiving/planAhead/long_distance_issues.html.

AARP. "My Parents—How Do I Know if They Need Help?" www.aarp.org/families/caregiving/caring_parents/a2003-10-27-caregiving-need help.

Alzheimer's Association. "Long-Distance Caregiving." www.alz.org/living_with_alzheimers_long_distance_caregiving.asp.

Eldercare Locator. "How Will I Know Mom and Dad Are Okay?" www.eldercare.gov/eldercare/Public/resources/fact_sheets/pdfs/INTOUCH_brochure.pdf.

Family Caregiver Alliance. "Handbook for Long-Distance Caregivers." www.caregiver.org/caregiver/jsp/content_node.jsp?nodeid=1034.

Mace, Nancy, and Peter Rabins. "When You Live Out of Town." In *The 36-Hour Day: A Family Guide to Caring for Persons with Alzheimer's Disease, Related Dementing Illnesses, and Memory Loss in Later Life,* 4th ed. Baltimore, Md.: The Johns Hopkins University Press, 2006.

MetLife. "Long Distance Caregiving." www.metlife.com/WPSAssets/305 20778401118179212VIFLong%20Dist%20Caregiving.pdf.

Morris, Virginia, and Robert M. Butler. "Home Away From Home." In *How to Care for Aging Parents.* New York: Workman Publishing, 2004.

National Association of Professional Geriatric Care Managers. "Find a Care Manager." http://caremanager.findlocation.com/?

National Institute on Aging. "So Far Away: Twenty Questions for Long-Distance Caregivers." www.nia.nih.gov/HealthInformation/Publications/LongDistanceCaregiving.

CHAPTER 20: THE 10 BEST QUESTIONS

Before Joining an Alzheimer's
Support Group

A little help is better than a lot of pity.

—Celtic proverb

Why join a support group? Because people in support groups understand; they've been there, done that, or are just learning how to cope with Alzheimer's disease like you are. Where else could you find a banker and a construction worker opening their hearts to each other?

An AD support group is defined as a group of people who meet on a regular basis with a trained group leader to discuss their feelings and fears about AD. Some support groups consist of persons with AD, others are solely for caregivers or adult children, some groups are mingled or focused on married couples, and still others meet only online in informal chat rooms.

People of all ages, races, and backgrounds who have been touched by AD share similar concerns, worries, and the effects of caregiver exhaustion. Just knowing your Tuesday night support group meeting is tomorrow might help you get through one more day of your loved one's temper tantrums and soiled diapers.

Alzheimer's support groups can be a wonderful outlet to:

- Connect with others who are going through the same thing
- Overcome feelings of isolation, fear, and being overwhelmed
- Get insider information on the best doctors, treatments, books, and Web sites

LINDA DANO SHARES HER STORY

After her father was diagnosed with the disease and she became his primary caregiver, Linda Dano, one of daytime television's most beloved stars, became a national spokesperson for AD.ID (Identify Alzheimer's Disease), a program that helped caregivers deal with their loved ones' suffering.

Now she says, "My biggest advice is to share all this responsibility. I didn't go to a group; I didn't go to therapy. I never said a word to anyone. I was in so much pain."

- Express confusing or frightening emotions in a safe environment
- Feel less helpless knowing where to get more help
- Learn more about Alzheimer's.

The Alzheimer's Association is the national leader in establishing local, face-to-face support groups as well as online groups. There are also numerous other online, community, and local AD support groups.

Ask yourself the following Best Questions first to decide if a support group is right for you. If so, use the second set of Best Questions in this chapter to ask others (the group leader or the local chapter of the Alzheimer's Association) as you seek more information about support groups. This two-step process will help you determine what you really want and then help you get there.

>>>THE 10 BEST QUESTIONS
to Ask Yourself *Before Joining a Support Group*
(for Caregivers)

1. Why do I want to join? What are my expectations and are they realistic?

Many people touched by Alzheimer's disease need a sounding board for their feelings and questions. But belonging to a support group also takes a commitment of your time and energy, which may already be stretched thin by your role as a primary caregiver.

2. Am I a fairly open or fairly private person?

There is no right-wrong answer here. Your honest self-assessment will clarify how well suited you'll be for a support group. Seek a one-on-one counselor if you want undivided attention, private consultations, or have really major issues, like a catastrophic family disaster in progress. If you are open, have an extroverted personality, or too few close by confidants and want to share your caregiving experiences, consider joining a support group.

3. Do I want an in-person group or an online group?

As you ponder this personal choice, the factors to consider are your access to in-person support groups, your available time, if you like the idea of 24/7 access to online chat buddies, and your preference for virtual hugs versus live-body hugs.

Elder Rage author Jacqueline Marcell advises, "Find both groups so you have options. Online groups are great when you are up all night with a sundowner and you just need to talk to someone. It's daylight in Australia and they have caregivers there, too."

4. Do I have a face-to-face support group conveniently located for me?

How you define "conveniently located" depends on your willingness to spend time belonging to a support group. "Convenient" to you might be within ten miles, while "convenient" for others is within fifty miles.

5. How comfortable will I be with this particular group?

If you aren't sure, proceed with caution while you give the support group a fair try. Some people prefer to be with people very similar to themselves, while others enjoy generic caregiver groups.

For example, Lorraine Biros, client services director of the Mautner Project, The National Lesbian Health Organization, suggests, "It's important for lesbian patients to find a lesbian support group."

6. How emotionally rocky has my caregiving experience been so far?

This quickie reality test helps you to assess your own emotional stability, to consider your personal resiliency, and to count how many close family members and friends you've been able to count on.

7. Realistically, will I be able to keep up with the meeting schedule based on my other responsibilities?

You may not have any energy left after caregiving or be able to leave your loved one alone at home. Maybe you're still working full time or have a troubled teenager, too. Sometimes a regular commitment to a support group becomes another new stressor instead of a life-changing experience.

8. Do I want my loved one, family members, or friends to accompany me to my support group meetings, join a separate support group, or not be involved at all?

Think about how much you need to discuss your loved one's problems, behaviors, and your other relationships. If relationships are your central discussion focus, you may do better in separate groups. Your answer also depends, of course, on your loved one's current AD stage.

Erma in Houston, Texas, recalls, "When my husband, Roger, joined an Alzheimer's support group and talked with other AD patients who were experiencing the same outbursts, he started to calm down. He finally understood he wasn't the only one."

9. How will I feel when the group members' loved ones die?

If you are dealing with MCI or early stage AD, later-stage caregivers may either inspire or depress you. Just consider this question before getting involved.

10. Is this going to be helpful and will I feel better each time I participate in this group?

Some of the best support groups refuse to be falsely cheerful and brush aside the harsh realities of caregiving. For a low-risk trial, find an online support or one buddy to confide in before launching a full-scale public soul-baring in a community forum of your friends and neighbors.

❯ The Magic Question

When I walk out of this group (or sign off from an online group), do I feel inspired to live my life more fully?

Make every moment of your life count. A support group should be more inspiring and uplifting than depressing and stressful. Chances are you already have enough of your own stress, so don't absorb anyone else's, too.

>>> THE 10 BEST QUESTIONS
to Ask Others *Before Joining an Alzheimer's Support Group*

1. Who leads the group? What is this person's background, formal training, and experience with Alzheimer's patients and their families?

A skillful and experienced group leader can make a huge difference in your enjoyment and benefits from a support group. Look for someone who has already gone through caring for an AD patient herself. The ideal group leader, or "facilitator," also has training in managing group dynamics and feelings.

THE QUESTION DOCTOR SAYS:

Find out how this group leader deals with confidentiality issues. You may be sensitive and not want your personal situation discussed outside of the support group.

---

2. What does the group talk about?

Most support groups share common problems and fears and laugh through their tears at the things their AD loved ones say and do. There should be a healthy blend of happiness, sadness, and complaints, not an overabundance of any single emotion or topic.

3. Which stages of Alzheimer's disease are the participants dealing with?

If you have choices, you might want a support group where all the participants share the same problems caused by their loved ones at similar stages in the disease. The most important thing is finding out what you have in common with the other participants.

4. Are the participants either AD patients or family members or are both in a mixed group?

Again, this factor may not matter to you or you may have limited choices. Just be aware that early stage AD patients may be less sympathetic to caregivers' woes and perspective than other caregivers—and vice versa.

5. What is the size and turnover of the group?

Lively discussions happen when groups have between six and fifteen attendees. People often drift in and out of support groups, depending on their other activities and responsibilities.

If you want more long-term stability, look for a well-established group of soul mates. It will save you having to retell your story and meet new people at each meeting.

6. Do any of the support group members socialize at times besides the regular group meetings?

You may not care about extended friendships outside of the support group. Just be aware of your own preferences ahead of time so you don't feel either forced or neglected by the other group members.

7. Who is sponsoring the group and why?

Most support groups are sponsored by nonprofit groups, including the Alzheimer's Association, hospitals, medical associations, and other community or religious organizations.

Be just a little more wary of online groups until you know more about who's behind them and what, if any, hidden motives they may have, such as promoting AD drugs or seeking volunteers to participate in a clinical trial.

8. Where does the group hold its meetings?

Face-to-face groups meet in hospital settings, members' homes, churches, community centers, and other community locations. If you are caring for an AD patient at home and need someone to stay with her while you're out, the convenience of the support group's location is likely to be important to you.

9. Is there an online component?

There are thousands of people in online groups discussing Alzheimer's at this very moment. Some groups chat on specific issues, like dealing with wandering or aggression, while others have less direction and structure.

10. What other alternatives to face-to-face support group meetings do I/we have?

Some burned-out caregivers need higher-level help than they initially realize. See chapter 17.

If you do, seek private counseling with a therapist, social worker, or a trusted religious or community leader. You may need help beyond what a support group can reasonably provide if you find yourself constantly angry and hurtful with your loved one.

❯ The Magic Question

How does the group leader protect participants' emotions and egos during group discussions?

There are certain risks to being an active member of a support group and sharing your true thoughts and feelings. A first-class group facilitator creates a safe place for people to share their stories and personal vulnerabilities.

The use of ground rules for discussion, such as, "All comments are welcome, but no personal attacks," defines the boundaries of acceptable discussion topics and behaviors and creates a safety net for all participants.

CONCLUSION

Seeking a support group may be the healthiest thing you can do for yourself. Even if you usually aren't a "group person" or can think of a million excuses, try it anyway. Alzheimer's disease is so devastating on caregivers because the progression is a long, slow decline, often lasting for years while the person is still being cared for at home.

As the primary caregiver, your usual coping methods just may not be adequate enough without a little help from your friends.

THE 10 BEST RESOURCES

Alzheimer's Association. "In My Community," Searchable database for local groups. www.alz.org/apps/findus.asp.

Alzheimer's Association. "Message Boards." www.alz.org/living_with_alz heimers_message_boards_lwa.asp.

Alzheimer's Association. "Support Groups and Dementia." Resource guide. www.alz.org/national/documents/SupportGroups_RL.doc.

Capossela, Cappy, and Sheila Warnock. *Share the Care: How to Organize a Group for Someone Who Is Seriously Ill.* New York: Simon & Schuster, 2004.

Carson, Nancy. "A Family Caregivers Support Group Guide." www.the familycaregiver.org/pdfs/SupportGrpGuide.pdf.

Children of Aging Parents. "A National Organization for Caregivers." www.caps4caregivers.org/.

Mace, Nancy, and Peter Rabins. "Getting Outside Help." In *The 36-Hour Day: A Family Guide to Caring for Persons with Alzheimer Disease, Related Dementing Illnesses, and Memory Loss in Later Life*, 4th ed. Baltimore, Md.: The Johns Hopkins University Press, 2006.

Mayo Clinic. "Support Groups: Find Information, Encouragement, and Camaraderie." www.mayoclinic.com/health/support-groups/MH00002.

Well Spouse Association (Canada). "Support Programs." www.wellspouse .org/index.php?option=com_content&task=section&id=8&Itemid=37.

Wellness Community. "Worldwide Locations." www.thewellnesscommu nity.org/corporate/facilities.php.

CHAPTER 21: THE 10 WORST QUESTIONS
to Ask People with Alzheimer's Disease

> The human race has one really effective weapon, and that
> is laughter.
>
> —Mark Twain

When coping with a loved one who has Alzheimer's disease, you have many reasons to be sad, stressed, or depressed. "Down days" are to be expected. Don't pretend to be cheerful when you're not. Be honest and talk about all your feelings, not just the cheerful ones.

On the other hand, humor is a powerful ally. Over the past decades, studies have found that humor can reduce physical pain, aid the immune system, and keep the brain alert. The message is simple: humor is healing. The medicinal power of laughter can fight your fear and uncertainty and help to lighten your caregiver's load. Most people with AD tend to retain their sense of humor and may be delighted to laugh along with you.

In his pioneering 1979 book *Anatomy of an Illness,* Norman Cousins asserted that "laughter therapy" cured him from a supposedly irreversible disease. "Nothing is less funny than being flat on your back with all the bones in your spine and joints hurting," he wrote. Cousins started watching old Marx Brothers films and TV's *Candid Camera* while still in the hospital. He discovered that ten minutes of genuine belly laughter had an anesthetic effect that allowed him to get two hours of pain-free sleep.

Welcome to the the Hall of Shame, the Worst Questions asked by well-meaning but clueless friends and family members of the primary caregiver. This chapter is a collection of those Worst Questions that caregivers hear from people who don't know what else to say or how to talk to someone with Alzheimer's disease or their caregiver.

>>> THE 10 WORST QUESTIONS
to Ask People with Alzheimer's Disease

1. Did I tell you about my grandmother, Nina, who had Alzheimer's and went totally mental in just two months?

One of the most universally despised and most common Worst Questions involves telling a long shaggy-dog story about someone else's experience with Alzheimer's, especially one with a tragic ending.

Nina has nothing to do with anything except maybe it's the only way the listener can relate to you at all. But in essence, a Nina story allows the listener to hijack your right to talk about your personal experience and feelings.

2. What did you (or your loved one) do to get Alzheimer's disease?

One of the most common misconceptions in our hyper health-conscious society is that somehow people cause or are responsible for their own diseases. No one knows with 100 percent certainty what causes most Alzheimer's cases. This Worst Question indicates a blame-the-victim mindset. Don't fall for it. It's not anyone's fault.

3. How long do you (or your loved one) have to live?

This innocent question reflects the asker's ignorance of AD complexity and the fact that many people with MCI or early stage AD can live several years relatively symptom free. Sometimes people just don't know what else to ask except to ask "time" questions—how long, how short, how often, etc.

4. Can you or your loved one still talk? Do you/does he remember my name?

Because most people are afraid of an Alzheimer's diagnosis but don't really understand the disease, they just can't imagine what it must be like. Some people may even act like the person with AD is from Mars or contagious. Reassure your family and friends and explain what level of language comprehension is reasonable to expect at this AD stage.

5. What are you so worked up about? Can't you just put him in a nursing home?

This awful question lacks any shred of sympathy, empathy, or understanding about what's involved and the complexities and hardships of caring for someone with AD.

It's the opposite of Worst Question 3 above. Instead of assuming a worst case scenario, now the asker has unconsciously assumed you'll automatically opt for long-term institutional care. The asker has also discredited your need to share your information or feelings that you might have been on the verge of talking about.

6. Do you remember where the buried treasure is?

OK, it's a bad joke. You can laugh at it ignore it, or take a swing at the other person, depending on your mood and the question asker's intent. There are lots of memory jokes out there.

7. Can your spouse still be romantic and have sex?

Coming from the right person, this can be a kind and caring question. The asker's motivation behind this question may be purely good-hearted and an invitation to talk. But if asked in a prying, inquisitive manner or by someone you aren't close to, this can also be an out-of-bounds question. The asker most likely really wants to know, "What's going on in your bedroom?"

THE QUESTION DOCTOR SAYS:

Caregivers and communication experts agree that open-ended questions that force "choice" responses may confuse someone with AD and put him on the spot. Using closed questions with simple yes or no answers is a better strategy.

When talking with someone with Alzheimer's, set a positive mood for interactions, keep good eye contact, avoid corrections or criticisms, focus on her feelings rather than logic or facts, use short, simple words, ask one simple question at a time, and wait patiently for responses.

Claudia Strauss, a communications instructor and author of *Talking to Alzheimer's*, suggests, "Whatever you do in communicating it's important to maintain the other person's dignity. When you ask questions that people can't answer, it affects their self-image. Our instinctive response is to use logic, but what works better is to validate their feelings, focus on what's happening in the present, and let questions about the past come from them, not you."

Here are some simple examples from Ms. Strauss and others on how to turn bad questions into better questions.

Bad Questions	Better Questions
(too vague or open ended for AD patients)	(closed questions with simple yes/no answers)
What TV programs do you like to watch?	Do you like to watch TV?
What are your favorite foods?	Does that taste good?
What do you want to wear today?	Do you want to wear your black pants or your tan pants today? (while holding up both pairs of pants)
What did you do yesterday?	Do you remember that time years ago when . . . ?

8. Does the poor little fellow want a cookie?

Please, no baby talk with people who have Alzheimer's disease. They are memory challenged, not three years old.

9. Can you hear me?

This question—especially shouted at the person with AD who is sitting next to you and has no hearing loss—doesn't make sense, but people ask it all the time anyway. Somehow we equate hearing with understanding, and deafness with mental retardation. Treat this person with as much respect as any other.

10. You mean *this*, don't you? Here, let me finish your sentence for you.

Many well-intentioned but impatient people rush to fill in the blanks when the person with AD is talking. This is especially frustrating for people with either early stage AD or MCI because it robs them of their chance to complete their thoughts—the ones that are still there but are just coming a little slower these days.

❯ The Magic Question

Did I tell you today how much I love you?

What a nice question to ask a person with short-term memory loss. Even if you already did say this today and your loved one has forgotten, now is a great time to say it again.

CONCLUSION

In order not to be offended by any of these Worst Questions, ask yourself, "Are these folks trying to upset me or are they trying to comfort me?" Usually the answer is "trying to comfort."

So instead of angry thoughts like, How can you possibly know what this is like for me?, focus on their sincerity in trying to be helpful. Then come up with some of your own Best Questions for small talk conversations and ask them to start over again.

Some caregivers choose to let their sense of humor take over and help them get through the worst time of their lives.

THE 10 BEST RESOURCES

Alzheimer's Australia. "Communication: Caring for Someone with Dementia." www.alzheimers.org.au/upload/HS2.1.pdf.

Association for Applied and Therapeutic Humor. "Humor Resources Archive." www.aath.org/archive.htm.

Cousins, Norman. *Anatomy of an Illness.* New York: W. W. Norton, 1979.

Family Caregiver Alliance. "Caregiver's Guide to Understanding Dementia Behaviors." www.caregiver.org/caregiver/jsp/content_node.jsp?nodeid=391.

Hodgson, Harriet. *Alzheimer's: Finding the Words, A Communication Guide for Those Who Care.* New York: John Wiley and Sons, 1995.

Klein, Allen. *The Courage to Laugh.* New York: Tarcher/Putnam Books, 1998.

Mayo Clinic. "Communicating Effectively with a Person Who Has Alzheimer's." www.mayoclinic.com/health/alzheimers/AZ00004.

Radin, Lisa. "Stages and Levels of Questioning." In *What If It's Not Alzheimer's: A Caregiver's Guide to Dementia.* Amherst, N.Y.: Prometheus Books, 2003.

Wooten, Patty. *Compassionate Laughter: Jest for Your Health*, 2nd. ed. Santa Cruz, Calif.: JestHealth, 2000.

Wooten, Patty. *Heart, Humor and Healing.* Santa Cruz, Calif.: JestHealth, 1994.

PART V:

Planning for the Future

Planning for the future plays a significant role in successful coping with life after a diagnosis of Alzheimer's disease. Advance planning should include making difficult decisions about driving, financial affairs, end-of-life legal concerns, and choosing hospice care. Each chapter in this section discusses the 10 Best Questions for one of these issues and offers practical advice along with the potential best answers.

Deciding when to retire from driving is particularly difficult for many AD patients and families, so there are two lists of Best Questions here. One is a checklist of the warning signs for declining driving skills and the other will guide your actual discussion with your loved one.

Many people, including caregivers, would rather bury their heads in the sand than face up to end-of-life financial and legal concerns. Once you've got your head back up and the sand is out of your ears, use these Best Questions to calm your fears, learn what your loved one's last wishes are, and empower yourself to make wise choices and decisions.

The book closes with a chapter on choosing hospice services. It's smart not to let your emotions at this difficult time make you especially vulnerable to overpaying for mediocre hospice care. You and your loved one deserve the very best.

CHAPTER 22: THE 10 BEST QUESTIONS
for Deciding When to Retire
from Driving

The best car safety device is a rearview mirror with a cop in it.

—Dudley Moore

After first hearing the shocking words "Alzheimer's disease," the next thought is often, "Car keys." There are few issues more important—or more contentious—after a diagnosis of mild, early stage AD or MCI than driving. These AD patients will often have sufficient cognitive functioning to adjust and stay behind the wheel.

Since the progression of Alzheimer's is gradual, unpredictable, and irreversible, everyone with AD eventually stops driving. The hard question is deciding *when* is the right time for the person to cut back or stop driving altogether. Even the experts can't agree. The Alzheimer's Association recommends a case-by-case approach, while the American Academy of Neurology suggests no further driving at any stage.

It isn't just AD patients who ultimately face driving retirement. It happens to everyone. All drivers who live beyond a certain age (even without mental impairments) must consider the dangers of continuing to drive. The statistics from the National Highway Traffic Safety Administration may surprise you. Drivers over seventy-five years old have a higher risk of being involved in a collision for every mile they drive than any other age group. They are nearly as accident prone as the riskiest sixteen- to twenty-four-year-old drivers. Older drivers involved in accidents have higher fatality rates than younger drivers.

But even when shown these facts along with the new dents on every side of his car, your loved one may still refuse to believe he's a bullheaded road menace. Many AD drivers fail to recognize their own declining driving abilities, especially if they live alone. Several studies have revealed that older drivers view their family members—especially their children—as the least credible people to discuss this topic with. Men are more likely than women to resist driving restrictions.

If you are a frustrated adult daughter, get outside help for your ornery father. His doctor is a good place to start since many states require doctors to notify the state's motor vehicle department routinely about AD/dementia diagnoses. The American Medical Association encourages doctors to discuss driving restrictions with their AD patients as a "retirement." It's important that the AD patient be included in the initial decision making to ensure better compliance with driving limitations now and later.

This chapter has two sets of Best Questions. First, if you are worried about your loved one's driving (or if you are the AD patient), ask *yourself* the initial set of questions to make a well-informed decision about how serious the problem is. These Best Questions are adapted from the lists of standard warning signs of driving trouble available from the Alzheimer's Association, AARP, and Hartford Financial Services Group Web sites.

Use the second set of Best Questions when you are talking with your loved one about his declining driving abilities. The assumption is that you or another reliable person has recently witnessed his driving and you have valid concerns. If the topic of surrendering the car keys is a hotly contested battleground in your family, these Best Questions will help you prepare for this discussion in advance. You may need several discussions or may have to pick and choose questions that will work well with your loved one.

Be sure to seek concurrence from your doctor or law enforcement officials on your driving decisions. The Alzheimer's Association and the AARP have extensive resources to help you decide wisely. When in doubt, don't drive.

>>> THE 10 BEST QUESTIONS
for Deciding When to Retire from Driving

1. Does the driver act increasingly nervous, afraid, confused, or angry while driving in routine road conditions?

These reactions often signal a decrease in your loved one's self-confidence as a driver. She may feel more uncomfortable behind the wheel but be reluctant to say anything for fear of losing her driving rights.

Other signs are increased agitation, confusion, or irritation while driving. An example is confusing simple dashboard controls or dials and then being defensive about it.

2. Do other drivers and passengers act nervous, afraid, or angry when your loved one is driving?

Is there a new pattern of other drivers angrily honking their horns or shaking their fists at your loved one in traffic? Has the driver recently received several warnings or traffic tickets issued by the police? Do friends and relatives seem increasingly reluctant to drive with your loved one? These are all important signs of unsafe driving.

3. Is the driver having frequent close calls or showing up with new dents and scrapes on the car?

Frequent near misses, new dents and scrapes on the car or garage walls, flattened mailboxes, and rubber marks on curbs and sidewalks are not normal and point to an unsteady, unsure driver.

4. Is the driver making slower decisions and showing poor judgment while driving?

Older people have impaired spatial skills and slower reaction times. This explains their poorly timed left-hand turns and frequent problems with maintaining or changing lane positions. Your loved one may misjudge traffic gaps at intersections, on the highway, and on entrance/exit ramps.

Other common judgment problems are waiting too long for a traffic break or impulsively pulling into oncoming traffic, failure to stop or yield in sufficient time, stopping in traffic for no apparent reason, and poor distance perception in general.

5. Is my loved one getting lost or confused even in her own neighborhood?

Getting lost in familiar places is a serious warning sign that should not be ignored.

6. Does my loved one have difficulty reading traffic signs, road signals, and dashboard controls?

Suddenly losing the ability to read common road signs or traffic signals, understand street names, see pavement markings, and comprehend the car's dashboard controls is not normal. A person with AD may try to cover up his confusion, but this is ultimately quite dangerous, especially coupled with his slowed reaction time.

7. Is my loved one disregarding standard rules of the road with increasing frequency?

Examples include changing lanes without signaling, running red lights and stop signs, and parking inappropriately in forbidden parking zones. Look especially for a strong contrast between your loved one's former good driving habits and his driving now, but don't overreact to one minor turn signal mistake.

8. Does she drive too fast or too slow for the traffic circumstances?

Driving at an inappropriate speed frequently indicates that the driver lacks full awareness of the general traffic flow and prevailing road conditions. Drivers with AD may try to compensate for confusion with overly aggressive or passive driving behaviors, or by dangerously riding the brakes.

9. Does my loved one become easily distracted or lose attention while driving?

Do not ignore indictors that the driver is becoming more easily distracted by routine traffic conditions or is having a hard time concentrating behind the wheel. AD drivers should not use cell phones while driving.

10. Does my loved one have any physical limitations, including vision, hearing, or flexibility problems, that are affecting his safety on the road?

Physical frailties can't be ignored when you're assessing his driving. Older drivers may have dangerously impaired vision or hearing conditions. Pay attention if your loved one complains he can't see the sides of the road when looking straight ahead.

Some older drivers find it hard to turn and look over their shoulder when backing up, changing lanes, and parking or take medications that may affect their driving safety.

❯ The Magic Question

How well can the driver react to multitasking demands and unexpected situations?

It's one thing to miss traffic signs or misjudge the speed for changing lanes. But it's another thing not to be able to handle multiple tasks or anticipate dangerous driving situations such as a parked truck that is blocking traffic, an ambulance with its lights flashing and siren on suddenly coming from behind, or a young boy on a wobbly bike riding too close to traffic. This diminished critical thinking ability is what official examiner's tests look for if a driver has been diagnosed with AD/dementia.

Being a good driver means being able to follow multiple instructions, concentrate, recall information, and perform divided-attention tasks. If someone is confused or forgetful, she may not respond appropriately to emergencies or fast-changing road conditions.

❯❯❯ THE 10 BEST QUESTIONS
to Discuss Retirement from Driving with Your Loved One

Discussing driving decisions with your loved one with AD may be one of the most difficult conversations you ever have. Most families and AD patients find themselves somewhere on a slippery slope between denying the problem, anger over lost independence and mobility, panic about a potential accident, and sadness about a reduced quality of life.

Because no two families or relationships are the same and each diagnosis of AD has its own unique progression, there are no easy answers (or questions) about when to stop driving. Caregivers and adult children can try to minimize stress and family frictions and reduce the driver's defensiveness by having a direct conversation and including the driver in the decision-making process.

Most experts believe this straightforward method works better than more devious tactics like stealing and hiding the car keys or pretending nothing is wrong. Keep in mind that many AD patients may think their driving abilities are unchanged despite clear warning signs to the contrary.

Frank, early discussions will help you to avoid major confrontations later. Luckily, giving up the car keys can be a gradual process rather than a dramatic, one-time event. Knowing what to say and being prepared for this tough conversation will increase the likelihood that your loved one has a safe and successful transition from being a driver to becoming a passenger.

1. Did you hear about the car accident in the news today?

This question is a conversation starter to get your loved one thinking about older drivers' accidents in general. If you get a grunted "yes" or "no" response, use a follow-up question like the next one.

2. Does it seem to you that traffic is getting worse and it's harder to drive?

This question can ease you into a general conversation about the worst driving conditions, like peak traffic or nighttime. Your goal here is for your loved one to volunteer willingly to give up driving during these most stressful conditions as the first stage to total driving cessation.

Family members can find common ground by sharing traffic horror stories and how to avoid difficult road conditions, construction sites, or changing traffic patterns.

3. Do you think other drivers are becoming more unpredictable? What can *you* do about it?

If someone is in denial about his own declining driving abilities, he may blame others, such as younger drivers. Listen closely to your loved one's answer as a window into his possible unspoken fears. As he answers the second question, listen for how proactive his response is ("I could slow down," etc.) or see if he thinks of himself more as an out-of-control victim. A victim mentality can be tougher to deal with because it may signal his lack of willingness to make appropriate changes.

4. How did Granddad stop driving?

The Hartford Institute for Geriatric Nursing suggests this question in its brochure "Family Conversations with Older Drivers" as an opportunity to learn more about your loved one's personal feelings and family history of driving.

5. What are your best qualities as a driver?

First let your loved one brag about his previously great driving record as a way to transition to tougher questions. You can thus minimize his defensiveness and move into a conversation that pinpoints the least hazardous driving trips, like simple errands, that he may still be able to do.

6. How has your driving changed since your diagnosis of AD/ dementia? What do you see as your most difficult driving challenges or concerns?

By tying these two direct questions together, you've let your loved one rightfully point to AD as the cause of his poorer driving in the recent past. Even if you encounter denial or resistance in his response, you've paved the way for a solution-seeking discussion in the next question. Try to be a nonjudgmental listener as he shares his driving fears and concerns about safety. If he's defiant, try asking this question again at another time.

7. What are other ways you can get around without driving?

If your loved one has early stage AD and can still reason fairly well, turn this discussion into a brainstorming session for solutions. Let her lead the way in finding her own alternatives to driving. Perhaps you can research public transportation ahead of time for the facts, but a smart strategy is let her self-discover her own solutions first.

Avoid being condescending or overly critical about any suggestions she makes. If she reacts to this question with confusion, anger, or defiance, you may need to be more direct. Be ready to spell out the available alternatives to driving, such as public transportation, bus routes, rides from friends, and hired drivers.

8. Which friends or other family members can provide rides at the times you require?

Most seniors prefer familiar family members and friends as their alternative drivers. This method is more social, comfortable, and safer for AD patients.

9. What programs offer rides and are available in your area?

Most regions have local ride programs through churches, synagogues, local government agencies, senior services, or other nonprofit groups. Ask in advance about passenger eligibility, schedules, routes, hours, payments, help with packages or wheelchairs, driver safety precautions, and preregistration requirements.

10. How would you feel if you hurt or killed someone?

Save this question as your extreme backup plan if all other questions or approaches fail to bring your defiant loved one to his senses about his driving. No one likes to be told he's a dangerous driver, and this is especially demeaning from an adult child or spouse.

If your loved one truly is no longer safe behind the wheel, then tell him so. If he won't listen to you, ask his doctor or police for guidance and support.

THE QUESTION DOCTOR SAYS:

Being well prepared is the best way to handle this difficult conversation. To prepare, keep a written record of your observations on the AD person's recent driving patterns to back up your concerns. But also accentuate the positive, be solution focused rather than blaming, and be ready to suggest viable transportation alternatives.

Use neutral phrases like "retirement from driving" and "becoming a passenger" to minimize your loved one's denial and sense of loss.

As the caregiver, you must also cope with your own feelings of anger, frustration, and guilt about depriving your loved one of his freedom to drive. Get in touch with your feelings as you prepare for an open, honest, and caring communication on this often sensitive topic.

❯ The Magic Question

What can you do in return for the people who give you rides?

If your loved one balks at this or worries about inconveniencing others as he starts to get more and more rides instead of driving himself, suggest things he can do in exchange for the rides, such as paying for the gas or weeding a friend's garden. This exchange may ease his guilt about imposing on others and helps to "even the score" by creating reciprocal relationships.

CONCLUSION

Driving and dementia don't mix. Caregivers need to be vigilant about observing driving behaviors, make well-informed decisions about how and when to intervene, and be sensitive to their loved one's negative reactions and need for mobility.

Don't avoid the warning signs of problem driving. Be direct and frank about your concerns. His life and well-being, as well as the lives and well-being of you and others, may be at stake.

THE 10 BEST RESOURCES

AARP. "Driver Safety." Source for finding driving skills classes for older drivers. www.aarp.org/families/driver_safety.

AARP. "When to Stop Driving." www.aarp.org/families/driver_safety/ driver_safetyissues/a2004-06-21-whentostop.html.

Alzheimer's Association. "Driving." www.alz.org/national/documents/ topicsheet_driving.pdf.

American Automobile Association Foundation for Traffic Safety. "Driver 55 Plus: Suggestions for Improvement." www.aaafoundation.org/quizzes/ index.cfm?button=driver55sugg.

American Medical Association. "How to Help the Older Driver." www .ama-assn.org/ama1/pub/upload/mm/433/help_older_driver.pdf.

American Medical Association. "Older Driver Safety." www.ama-assn.org/ ama/pub/category/8925.html.

Eldercare Locator. "Choices for Mobility Independence: Transportation Options for Older Adults." www.eldercare.gov/Eldercare/Public/about/ Trans%20Options%20Panels.pdf.

The Hartford. "At the Crossroads: Family Conversations About Alzheimer's Disease, Dementia and Driving." www.thehartford.com/alzheimers/brochure.html.

The Hartford. "Warning Signs for Older Drivers Worksheet." www.thehartford.com/talkwitholderdrivers/worksheets/warningsigns2.pdf.

Seniordrivers.org. "Giving Up the Keys: For Families and Individuals." www.seniordrivers.org/notdriving/notdriving.cfm.

CHAPTER 23: THE 10 BEST QUESTIONS
for a Caregiver's Financial Health

> I was alarmed at my doctor's report. He said I was sound
> as a dollar.
>
> —Ronald Reagan

As the caregiver of someone with Alzheimer's disease, you may not want to spend your energy on financial matters just now. Maybe you basically dislike handling money. Whatever your financial status is, think of this diagnosis as a wake-up call to get more financially savvy.

Alzheimer's treatment and care can be costly. According to Consumer Reports, for example, homes that had taken in a parent added seven thousand dollars or more to their household expenses. These costs included home remodeling and higher food, utility, and transportation expenses, in addition to the dependent parent's medical and care costs.

Your financial difficulties won't be solved easily, but having a heart-to-heart talk with yourself is a great first step for getting and staying healthy financially. The following Best Questions are written for caregivers because the burden of financial management often falls on them.

These questions also work well for the person with early stage AD or MCI and for adult children and their parents, married couples, or partners with pooled income to discuss together. This chapter should not be used as a substitute for professional financial or tax advice.

> **THE QUESTION DOCTOR SAYS:**
>
> Start your financial discussions early. Ideally, you want your loved one to participate in financial planning as much as possible. Be aware that the rate of cognitive decline is unpredictable and differs for each Alzheimer's patient.
>
> These discussions will give you a concrete plan that can address potentially troubling situations before they become crises. Some families say that advanced planning is actually a stress reducer because they felt more in control afterward and made better-informed decisions.

〉〉〉THE 10 BEST QUESTIONS
for a Caregiver's Financial Health

1. How well organized are my/your/our personal financial papers, accounts, and records?

Careful financial planning starts with putting in one place all the information you'll need. Find out now before memory slips away where documents are stored. Request access to passwords, account numbers, safety deposit boxes and get the names of financial advisors. In particular, make sure you have full and complete access to bank accounts.

Important financial documents include:

- Bank and brokerage account information
- Birth certificates
- Deeds, mortgage papers, or ownership statements
- Insurance policies
- Monthly or outstanding bills
- Pension and other retirement benefit summaries
- Rental income paperwork

- College scholarship and grant money for your children
- Social security information
- Stock and bond certificates

2. What are my/your/our financial assets?

It's important to establish how much money your loved one has in cash, investments, insurance plans, and retirement benefits. As the caregiver, you need to consider carefully the upcoming medical and care expenses. A diagnosis of AD often calls for a change in your investment and savings strategies.

As the caregiver, you need to have financial plans in place in case something happens to you because your role in providing financial support is more important than ever. Cicily Carson Maton, a Certified Financial Planner in Chicago, says, "Emotional distress and lack of financial knowledge will impair your ability to make decisions." A financial advisor experienced in helping people with life-threatening diseases can help you make decisions and adjustments.

Possible sources of income and assets include:

- Stocks
- Bonds
- Savings accounts
- Real estate
- Reverse mortgage to convert home equity into income
- Personal property, such as jewelry or artwork

3. What are the estimated long-term total costs for my loved one's care?

Costs can run high. The Alzheimer's Association's research revealed that families spend an average of $175,000 in care over the course of the disease. Housing costs in particular can have a major impact.

To plan a long-term budget, list the expenses you may face in the future, such as:

- Adult day care
- Care in a long-term care facility (nursing home, etc.)
- In-home health care services
- Prescription drugs
- Treatment for Alzheimer's and other medical problems associated with aging
- Hospice care

In addition, you'll have everyday financial responsibilities, including paying mortgage, utility, credit card, health insurance, and other bills. You may have to prepare taxes or household accounts for your loved one, too.

There are various financial services that may help defray the costs if you are eligible. Consult with a knowledgeable financial advisor. Keep in mind that medical costs will continue to rise over time as your loved one's condition worsens and all medical costs continue to rise annually.

4. Do I/we need help from a professional financial advisor?

This may be a question you can't answer without first investigating the services and costs of financial advisors. You may want at least one session to help you identify potential resources, tax deductions, and how to avoid bad investment decisions.

Paul Yurachek, a Certified Financial Planner with Ameriprise Financial, says, "When people are aging, it creates a whole new set of issues, especially if there's a spouse involved. As financial advisors, we try to alleviate their concerns about money."

Financial planner Cicily Carson Maton advises clients about other options. She says, "If you didn't have any financial planning in place or didn't have a financial advisor prior to your diagnosis, reach out to those people around you whom you trust and ask for their help. You need to put together a team. Maybe this financial team will be your family members, maybe a trusted friend or a minister."

5. How do I find a well-qualified financial advisor?

Look for a Certified Financial Planner with proven experience in dealing with Alzheimer's patients or other terminal illnesses. As you are calling around, ask for the advisors' specific services, if they sell products (be wary), their personal philosophy on financial planning (conservative, aggressive, etc.), whom exactly you'll be working with, if charges are by the hour, flat fees, or commissions, and a written list of their services and charges.

You can also contact your local Alzheimer's Association office for its referrals of qualified financial advisors, accountants, and legal experts who understand the financial impact of Alzheimer's disease.

Norman Berk, a Certified Financial Planner at Professional Asset Strategies, in Birmingham, Alabama, suggests you first ask yourself, " 'How realistic am I and do I need outside financial help to assess my finances?' The typical response is, 'I don't need help,' but most people actually do. This is especially true for caregivers who may be very unrealistic about financial matters." Then you'll be ready for your first meeting with a financial advisor.

6. What are my/your/our insurance options?

Look at all your insurance options, including health care coverage, Medicare, disability, long-term care, and life insurance plans. Understanding these policies now can save you time and money later.

A primary concern is your health insurance. Norman Berk says, "One of your early questions should be what your health insurance coverage is and its portability. Once you know what you are faced with, you need an understanding with your insurance company on what it does or doesn't cover. This will impact your other decisions."

Since most people with Alzheimer's disease are sixty-five or older, health coverage is usually obtained through Medicare. But the fine print and loopholes for Medicare coverage are worth investigating now so you won't be caught by surprise. For example, Medicare provides some payment for in-home health care under certain conditions, does not cover custodial long-term nursing home care, and may cover hospice care. You can get help from your State Health Insurance Assistance Program (SHIP) at 800-272-3900 or visit www.medicare.gov/contacts/static/allStateCon tacts.asp.

Disability insurance may pay some costs if your loved one had a prediagnosis insurance plan in place. Some people have long-term care insurance policies, but these are also tricky. Make sure you understand exactly what's covered, when payments will begin, tax implications, and any maximum lifetime payout stipulations. After a diagnosis of AD, it is usually not possible to buy disability and long-term care insurance.

Life insurance or veterans insurance can be valuable sources of cash or collateral for getting a loan. Some policies offer accelerated death benefits, which pay insurance benefits before death if the person is not expected to live more than six to twelve months.

7. What are my options and eligibility for government assistance programs?

The primary government health care program for people over sixty-five is Medicare. In addition, the person with Alzheimer's and his family, if eligible, may qualify for public programs that support long-term care, such as:

- Social Security Disability Insurance (SSDI)
- Supplemental Security Income (SSI)
- Veterans' benefits
- Tax deductions and credits
- Care credit

SSDI is for workers under age sixty-five who can prove they are unable to work and have a disability that will last at least one year or result in death. Family members may also receive SSDI benefits. The Social Security Administration is slow in making eligibility decisions, so apply sooner rather than later. Be prepared to appeal an initial rejection.

SSI guarantees a monthly income for people age sixty-five or older who are disabled and have limited incomes. Medicaid pays for medical care for people with very low incomes and for long-term care for people who have used up their own money. Veterans may qualify for health and long-term care benefits. There are also various tax and care credits available. Check with www.benefitscheckup .org, the Veterans Administration, or your local Alzheimer's Association for more details.

8. What work-related salary and benefits are available to me/us/ you as potential income?

It's often possible for persons with early stage Alzheimer's or MCI to continue working for a while. The Americans with Disabilities Act (ADA) offers limited protection to those employed people with Alzheimer's, such as requiring the employer to offer a less demanding job, or to make reasonable accommodation for their disability.

If your loved one believes she's been unfairly treated, it's possible to file a discrimination claim under ADA. Check with a benefits specialist or her employer.

Other work-related benefits are available under the Family and

Medical Leave Act (FMLA), which allows the caregiver to take up to twelve weeks of unpaid leave each year to provide caregiving with a guarantee of keeping her job upon return. Some employers offer paid time off, flexible work schedules, or part-time employment. If the person with AD is your dependent under tax rules, you may be able to use a workplace flexible spending account to cover part of your out-of-pocket medical expenses or dependent care costs.

Retirement plans include individual retirement accounts (IRAs) and annuities. Benefits from retirement/pension plans can be important sources of income before retirement age if the worker is defined as disabled under the plan's guidelines. A person with AD may be able to withdraw money from his IRA or employee-funded retirement plan before age 59½ without penalties. Social Security benefits are also available before retirement age in some cases.

9. What income tax breaks might I quality for?

It makes sense to learn about the income tax deductions and credits that you may qualify for if your loved one is considered your dependent for tax purposes. For example, you may be eligible for deductions on medical expenses and or receive dependent care credits on your tax returns.

Deductible expenses may include nursing services, home improvements like grab bars, in-home care such as physical therapy, residential care, and expenses for personal care items. To claim federal income tax deductions, caregivers must first seek certification of justifiable expenses by a licensed health care practitioner.

State tax credits vary by state, with forty-one states providing help with the costs of private care for Alzheimer's patients. Each state has different qualifying expenses and different credit amounts. Contact your state department of revenue.

If you pay someone to care for your loved one so you can keep your job, you may be entitled to the Child and Dependent Care Credit. Be sure to keep careful records of all medical and care expenses for tax purposes.

10. What free or low-cost community services are available to help me?

Take advantage of the community services right under your nose. These services may include respite care, support groups, home-delivered meals, hospital social workers, adult day care (see chapter 13), friends or family members, and transportation services.

Your local religious organization may organize help on your behalf. Perhaps your family will pool resources to help pay for care. Think creatively about other ways to raise money or find financial resources.

❭ The Magic Question

Do I need to increase my own life insurance or disability insurance?

You may need to increase your own life insurance or disability insurance to provide a financial safety net for you and your loved one.

One important long-range financial goal when you are caring for someone with Alzheimer's is to avoid going broke. Consider what financial planning you need in place in case something happens to you. Having money in reserve in a rainy day fund is critical.

Cicily Carson Maton says, "Most financial planners say you need to have a cushion of three to six months' finances for living expenses in some kind of cash account that you can readily draw on." Ask yourself how close you are to meeting this financial goal with your own emergency funds.

CONCLUSION

Facing Alzheimer's as a caregiver is difficult and emotionally wrenching. Caring for a loved one—either your spouse or aging parent—often severely stretches your financial resources as well, especially when you consider the value of lost wages and retirement plan savings.

Coming to grips with financial realities soon after the initial diagnosis of AD helps families to confront the tough questions about future medical and care costs.

Planning ahead safeguards you against making poor decisions and gives you extra time to find financial resources, such as federal programs or employer-based benefits, that you otherwise may overlook.

THE 10 BEST RESOURCES

Administration on Aging. "Health Insurance Counseling." www.aoa.gov/eldfam/Elder_Rights/Health_Counseling/Health_Counseling.asp.

Alzheimer's Association. "Financial Matters." www.alz.org/living_with_alzheimers_financial_matters.asp.

Alzheimer's Association. "Medicare and Medicaid." www.alz.org/living_with_alzheimers_medicare_and_medicaid.asp.

Alzheimer's Association. "Money Matters: Helping the Person with Dementia Settle Financial Issues." www.alz.org/national/documents/brochure_moneymatters.pdf.

Alzheimer's Association. "Taxes and Alzheimer's Disease." www.alz.org/national/documents/brochure_taxes.pdf.

H.E.L.P. "Financial Issues." www.help4srs.org/finance/finintro.htm.

Medicare. "State Health Insurance Assistance Program (SHIP) Contact Information." www.medicare.gov/contacts/static/allStateContacts.asp.

MetLife. "Medicare and Medicaid Programs—The Basics." www.metlife.com/FileAssets/MMI/MMISYCMedicareandMedicaid2007.pdf.

National Council on Aging. "BenefitsCheckUp." Click on "Find More Benefits Programs" for questionnaires that will help you find the benefit programs you qualify for. www.benefitscheckup.org.

Social Security Administration. "Online Social Security Handbook." www .ssa.gov/OP_Home/handbook/ssa-hbk.htm.

CHAPTER 24: THE 10 BEST QUESTIONS

to Settle Legal Issues at the End of Life

> Our bodies are our gardens to which our wills are
> gardeners.
>
> —William Shakespeare

One of the most difficult issues after a diagnosis of Alzheimer's disease for patients, caregivers, and their families is dealing with legal issues and end-of-life decisions. Legal issues, such as organ donation and funeral planning, often also have strong emotional aspects that few people like to think about.

However, most patients and their families who settle their legal affairs in advance believe that having these documents and decisions in place, along with a clear understanding of the person's wishes about the use of life-prolonging treatments, makes it much easier for everyone later. The caregiver isn't overwhelmed with the stress of making urgent, life-or-death decisions without clear guidelines. The person with AD is confident her last wishes will be respected. The attending doctors can recommend treatments matched to the patient's values and desires.

As an example of what happens for many families, daytime television star Linda Dano shares her own painful experience. "If I had really found out what my father had wanted before I agreed to his feeding tube, really pursued it, I wouldn't be consumed with this guilt I will have until the day I die and can apologize to my father in person."

Getting your legal ducks in a row quickly is very important. Many of the necessary legal decisions should be made directly by the person with AD—and before the disease has robbed him of his cognitive abilities.

If you delay these discussions and decisions, you run the risk that the person with AD will be seen as legally incompetent in the eyes of the law. The disease robs people of the ability to think clearly and make decisions. If this happens before legal affairs are settled, the caregiver/family has the additional burden and expense of establishing a legal guardianship (also called a conservatorship).

Your doctor can help you get started by providing guidance on your loved one's medical condition, treatment options, procedures, and a discussing with you about what could happen in various medical situations later on. Your doctor may also be able to supply you with the necessary paperwork or suggest other resources such as a hospital, specialized attorney, or the local Alzheimer's Association chapter.

Caregivers can ask themselves the following Best Questions as a checklist for key end-of-life legal issues. These questions also work well for the person with AD to ask himself or for everyone to discuss together in family meetings. The more prepared you can be ahead of time, the easier these tough decisions will be, and you will be more confident that you are doing the right thing.

One word of caution: This chapter should not be used as a substitute for professional legal advice.

THE QUESTION DOCTOR SAYS:

Start these discussions early. Set a personal or family goal of having all the necessary legal documents signed by a certain date. It may take several family meetings to settle the final details. Plan a celebration afterward to reward yourselves for meeting your goal.

>>> THE 10 BEST QUESTIONS
to Settle Legal Issues at the End of Life

1. Am I clear about my loved one's personal preferences (also called an "advance directive") regarding the use of life-prolonging treatments?

An **advance directive** is defined as a written document or series of forms that indicate your preferences for medical treatment, end-of-life decisions, and the person who can make decisions for you if you are incapacitated. Most legal experts recommend that everyone have such a document.

Advance directives are based on the principle of a person's right to die with dignity. You express in advance how much or how little you want done for you at the point in time when you become incapacitated and can no longer speak, and make your wishes clear.

All federally funded health care facilities are required by law to ask if you have an advance directive or offer you appropriate information on creating one. The laws about advance directives vary from state to state; a lawyer may be useful but is not required for completing an advance directive. You can withdraw or revoke your advance directive at any time you choose.

There are two types of advance directives, a living will and a medical power of attorney. Each of these is discussed separately below.

2. Does my loved one have a living will? If so, do I have a copy? Do I fully understand it?

A **living will** states your preferences for medical care if you are unable to make your own decisions or cannot communicate. It is called a "living will" because it takes effect while you are still alive and deals only with your medical care, not the distribution of your property. A living will tells your family and health care providers

---

THREE MORE BEST QUESTIONS

To help you make these hard decisions, consider three follow-up questions:

1. What situations (such as extreme pain or weakness) would be so bad that I/my loved one would not want to prolong my/his life?
2. What medical treatments are acceptable on a temporary basis (such as to recover from an illness) but are not acceptable permanently?
3. What medical treatments are undesirable under any circumstances?

---

what type of life-prolonging treatments you want, such as your preferences for artificial nutrition and hydration through an IV line or tube, and what to do in case you reach a persistent vegetative state or permanent coma without hope of recovery.

This document's whole purpose is to help people die with dignity. It also protects the doctor and hospital from liability for withdrawing or limiting life support.

Most states have their own forms, and each form differs slightly. In general, a living will must be signed in the presence of two witnesses and notarized. You may want to have this document prepared by a lawyer so there will be no question later about your or your loved one's mental competency at the time the document was signed.

A **do not resuscitate (DNR) order** is a separate document that instructs medical personnel not to perform life-saving treatments (such as putting the patient on a ventilator) or other heroic measures to revive you if your heart stops or if you stop breathing.

As the caregiver, make sure you have clear access to this document and you fully understand your loved one's desires.

3. Does my loved one have a durable medical power of attorney for health care?

A **durable medical power of attorney** is a signed, dated, witnessed, and notarized document that names another person, usually a spouse, adult child, or close friend, as your substitute decision maker to make future medical decisions on your behalf if you are no longer capable of thinking or speaking. This person is called an "agent," "proxy," or "surrogate."

Most regular power of attorney documents become invalid with mental incapacity. In contrast, this document is "durable" because it continues after the person becomes legally mentally incapacitated. A durable power of attorney document can contain highly detailed instructions stating the scope of the agent's actions and specifying when the durable power of attorney goes into effect. For example, the agent can decide if the person will end life at home or in a facility, choose or refuse certain treatments or life support, or become an organ donor.

The agent should understand the person's needs and values and be someone who is calm under pressure and flexible enough to adapt to quickly changing circumstances. Some people also appoint an alternate agent as a backup. State laws may differ slightly.

4. Does my loved one have a durable power of attorney for finances?

A separate document called a **durable power of attorney for finances** designates an individual to be your agent or proxy for financial decisions. Similar to a medical power of attorney, this document specifies who can make financial decisions on your behalf in case you can no longer think clearly or communicate your wishes.

A durable power of attorney for finances can provide AD patients and their families with flexibility in managing financial matters. It can also help you avoid the need for court conservatorship or the judicial oversight of your financial affairs.

Chicago-based Certified Financial Planner Cicily Carson Maton states, "A power of attorney is very important to pay your bills and take care of your affairs if you are incapacitated and can't do it. You need a surrogate to make decisions for you, a person that you trust. This is vital."

Longtime caregiver and author Patricia Callone advises from her firsthand experience, "It's important from the very beginning that the family knows who will have the durable power of attorney and who will handle the finances for care."

5. Is my loved one's will up-to-date? Does it accurately reflect his wishes about the disposition of his property?

A **will** controls what happens to your property after you die. If you or your loved one doesn't have a will, take the universal advice of legal professionals and get one written, regardless of the size of the estate. Making a will lets your loved one choose what happens to his property and belongings after he dies.

The person also determines the care of dependent children and pets with his will. A will can spell out specific gifts, create trusts to manage the estate, and provide funeral and burial instructions. Making a will helps the surviving beneficiaries, family, and friends because it simplifies their lives when they are dealing with the estate after your passing. Having a will in place minimizes surviving children's petty squabbles over possessions and inheritances.

Experts believe that a will is especially important to have for a person with newly diagnosed Alzheimer's disease. Move quickly to create a will or make any changes to an existing will because your loved one must be deemed legally capable (have "testamentary capacity") for the will to be considered valid.

6. Does my loved one want to have a living trust document?

In a separate financial planning document called a **living trust,** a grantor (either you or your loved one) creates a trust and designates a person to serve as the trustee. The trustee follows the trust's terms after the grantor dies. The trustee manages assets for the trust's beneficiary and has a legal, enforceable fiduciary duty toward the beneficiary.

Living trusts are often used because they may allow assets to be passed to heirs without going through probate. A living trust can encompass a wide range of properties, provides a detailed plan for property disposition upon the grantor's death, and avoids the expense and delay of probate for wills. However, beneficiaries do not save on federal estate or state inheritance taxes. Talk with your financial planner or tax consultant for more advice.

7. Has my loved one spelled out her funeral wishes in enough detail that I understand what she wants?

Many people don't like to talk about or think about their own funerals. But most caregivers are grateful for getting clear instructions from their loved ones now, even though it may be several years until the disease's end stage. Planning for death can provide a sense of peace and help reduce anxiety or a sense of urgency.

However, prepaid funerals are *not* a smart idea, according to a 2001 study by *Consumer Reports*. This report states, "Paying today for the *promise* of services and merchandise delivered years from now is always an iffy proposition for the buyer." The drawbacks include requirements for paying the full amount in advance, inflexibilities for making casket or other changes later, and huge hidden fees.

The best advice is to do all the preplanning, including choosing burial plots, monuments, pallbearers, religious institutions, and the funeral service details, such as photos, music, and speakers, without prepaying large sums of money now.

8. Does my loved one want to write an ethical will?

An **ethical will** is a popular but not legally binding document that a dying person writes to share his end-of-life wisdom and lessons learned over a lifetime. For someone with early stage AD or MCI, writing an ethical will can provide an opportunity to reflect on life's meanings, share personal values, hopes, and thoughts, tell favorite stories, finalize unfinished business, and pass down important information about the family's history, culture, and relationships.

A similar idea is to audio- or videotape the person with early stage AD telling her life story, perhaps while reminiscing over old family photo albums or with other family members during the holidays. Many families later cherish these recordings as a way of preserving their family's history and keeping a positive memory of the AD patient before the onset of memory and behavioral changes from late-stage disease.

As Dr. Hamilton Beazley, the author of the book *No Regrets: A Ten-Step Program for Living in the Present and Leaving the Past Behind,* says, "The best questions at the end of life focus attention on what's important rather than what's urgent."

9. Do I/we need help from a legal professional?

Most experts suggest families seek the help of an experienced elder-law attorney. Choose one who is knowledgeable about the kinds of legal decisions you are facing and especially about the legal implications of an Alzheimer's diagnosis. Understanding how mental competency is legally defined can be very important.

Laws vary by state. An attorney can help interpret your state's laws as they apply to your circumstances, will understand your entitlements under Medicare laws, and can make suggestions on how the patient's last wishes can be carried out.

Changes in circumstances, such as a divorce, death in the family, relocation, or new grandchildren or stepchildren, can mean that an existing will needs revision. There are other legal documents that you may feel more secure about if they are prepared by a professional. A legal expert may be able to suggest ways the caregiver can protect her assets and avoid personal bankruptcy later on.

If you can't afford legal assistance, ask your local Alzheimer's Association about no- or low-cost legal aid in your community. It's also possible (although not recommended) to create your own legal documents using templates or forms available at bookstores, libraries, or online.

10. How well organized are my/his legal papers, accounts, and records?

Look around your home office or in your file cabinet and assess how many of these legal documents you currently have, how many you need, and how well organized your or your loved one's records are.

Here is a checklist summary of generally recommended documents; the documents you need may differ depending on your personal circumstances.

- Contact details for legal representatives/attorneys
- Do not resuscitate orders
- Durable financial power of attorney
- Durable medical power of attorney
- Ethical will
- Legal guardianship papers
- Living trust
- Living will
- Preferences for funeral arrangements

- Title to cemetery plot
- Trust documents
- Will (include the name and contact information for the will's executor and the will's precise location)

› The Magic Question

What other legal issues need to be settled before my loved one's mental capacity is further impaired?

Another way of asking this question is, "What am I unclear about?" or "What's missing?" in your legal planning.

You need to ask yourself and your loved one some version of this question as soon as possible to avoid unpleasant or costly surprises later on. Examples of discussions you may not have had yet include decisions about stepchildren or children from a former marriage, desires about organ or tissue donations, and who should inherit family heirlooms such as your grandmother's wedding ring.

CONCLUSION

Unfortunately, it is too easy to delay asking these legal Best Questions—until it's too late. Most people don't want to think about this subject, but when the time comes to make difficult decisions, they are glad they had planned well in advance.

As the caregiver or the early stage AD patient, you may need time to consider your legal options and end-of-life wishes. Just remember the patient's ability to contribute meaningfully will decline over time. In addition, you need to be clear on the legal definition of "mentally competent" for people with Alzheimer's disease.

THE 10 BEST RESOURCES

AARP. "AARP Legal Counsel for the Elderly: Background." www.aarp
.org/makeadifference/gettinghelp/articles/icebackground.html

Administration on Aging. "Senior Legal Hotline Directory." www.aoa
.gov/eldfam/elder_rights/legal_assistance/SRdirclient.pdf.

Aging with Dignity. "Five Wishes." www.agingwithdignity.org/5wishes
.html.

Alzheimer's Association. "Legal Plans: Assisting the Person with Dementia in Planning for the Future." www.alz.org/national/documents/
brochure_legalplans.pdf.

ElderLawAnswers. Home page. www.elderlawanswers.com/index.asp.

Elder Law Resource Center. "Resources." elderlawresourcecenter.com/
resources.html.

MetLife. "Legal Matters." www.metlife.com/FileAssets/MMI/MMISYC
LegalMatters2007.pdf.

National Academy of Elder Law Attorneys. "Locate an Elder Law Attorney." http://naela.ebiz.uapps.net/solutionsite/Default.aspx?tabid=148.

Nolo. "Financial Powers of Attorney." www.nolo.com/resource.cfm/cat
ID/4D6845C7-364F-4C75-BCD09E399AC12F0F/309/292/166.

Nolo. "Wills and Estate Planning." www.nolo.com/resource.cfm/catID/
FD1795A9-8049-422C-9087838F86A2BC2B/309.

CHAPTER 25: THE 10 BEST QUESTIONS
for Choosing Quality Hospice Care

Shared joy is a double joy; shared sorrow is half a sorrow.
—Swedish proverb

Hospice care is the end-of-life medical, psychological, and spiritual support provided by health professionals and volunteers. The goals of hospice care are to help people die with peace and dignity, control pain and disease symptoms (called "palliative care"), and support the family. In the United States, early hospice programs began in the 1970s as small, voluntary operations. However, the last ten years have seen a dramatic increase in hospice providers, with many today operated by large for-profit corporations.

Usually, hospice is sought at the point that death seems imminent. Care is often in the dying person's home and without aggressive interventions to prolong life. Hospice care is also available at hospice centers, hospitals, and in nursing homes. Hospice is a concept or way of dying more than a specific place.

Ask your doctor, hospital social worker, geriatric care manager or nurse, or friends for their recommendations for hospice providers. This task can easily slip to the back burner of busy caregivers. Make an appointment with yourself to check out hospices sooner rather than later. As you visit different hospices with your Best Questions in hand (or when hospice representatives come to meet you in your home), have a family member or friend with you for moral support, to help you listen, and to assess your choices.

The quality of hospice varies significantly from one hospice provider to another and across geographical regions. In most communities, you'll have a choice of hospices.

Many people don't understand or don't think about using hospice services. The following Best Questions will help you decide if hospice care is desirable for your loved one, and if so, help you to find a top-quality hospice provider.

>>> THE 10 BEST QUESTIONS
for Choosing Quality Hospice Care

1. How do I know whether or not hospice care is a good fit for my loved one and my family? What are your eligibility requirements?

You may still be uncertain whether you want hospice care or you may not fully understand what it involves. Take this opportunity of talking with a hospice expert to learn more. Be silent for now and just let this person educate you. Find out what hospice care involves, its advantages, and the costs so you can make a well-informed decision.

Ask about eligibility requirements before asking any other questions. Most hospices accept patients with a life expectancy of six months or less who have a referral from their personal doctor. Some hospices require a designated family caregiver as a condition of admission. Inquire if their policy is flexible enough to accommodate your needs.

2. Is your hospice service licensed, bonded, and accredited?

Licensing requirements vary by state. Only forty-three states require hospices to be licensed. Check with your state's health department or the Hospice Patients Alliance Web site for your state's regulatory requirements (www.hospicepatients.org/state-hosp-reg-urls.html).

Having in-home workers licensed and bonded is the equivalent of insurance protection against any potential legal problems. Find out about volunteers' status, too.

THE QUESTION DOCTOR SAYS:

Listen for this representative's unspoken attitude behind her presentation. The ideal presentation combines detailed, factual information wrapped up in soothing empathy and compassionate words.

Ask yourself, Does she respond well to my questions? Is she willing or resentful about explaining hospice care to me? Does she seem genuinely interested in helping me and my loved one or is she just going through the motions?

As with home care agencies, hospice accreditation is voluntary. If a hospice is nationally accredited by The Joint Commission or another formal accrediting organization, this is a reliable indicator that the hospice is committed to providing top-quality care and service. State Medicare-certified hospices have met federal minimum requirements for a basic level of patient care and management.

3. How does your hospice select and train employees? What is your typical patient-to-caregiver ratio?

Ask about the typical employee profile (background, education, hands-on hospice experience). Listen for specific hospice and Alzheimer's training programs.

Here are more follow-up questions about employees:

- What is your staff turnover rate?
- Do you conduct full criminal background checks on all your prospective employees and volunteers? (Make sure volunteers are also checked.)
- How many employees have you fired for any reason in the last two years?

Smaller patient-to-caregiver ratios are better because the hospice caregivers will have more time and energy to devote to your family. If the ratio seems too high, ask about volunteers' availability and credentials.

4. Does a nurse, social worker, or therapist conduct a preliminary assessment for our suitability for hospice? Are family members included?

You want a needs assessment that is conducted in your home and not over the telephone. This assessment should include consultations with your loved one's doctors, other medical professionals (nursing home staff, etc.), and family members.

Dale Johnson, an executive director for The Joint Commission and responsible for accrediting hospice services says, "It's very delicate situation and you want an organization that is super-sensitive to your needs."

5. What specific services can we expect or request?

As part of this question, you want to know:

- How quickly can the provider initiate services?
- Is there a written description of available services?
- How do they manage patients' pain?
- Do they have a copy of a patient bill of rights for me?
- Do they provide any medical equipment, and if so, at what cost? Are caregivers trained in its use?

In the case of inpatient care services at a hospice facility, make sure you understand what services are provided and what will happen if your loved one no longer needs this service but isn't able to return home.

If your loved one is in a nursing home, ask if the nursing home contracts with this hospice provider. If so, ask if the hospice provides the same level of service in a nursing home as it does in a home setting. Before you accept their "yes" answer, ask for an example or more explanations. Their answer should confirm that they provide around-the-clock nursing services beyond normal care, spiritual and emotional support, family counseling, coordination with the patient's doctor, and pain management.

6. Does your hospice develop a written plan of care for each new patient? If so, are the caregiver, family, and patient involved in this process?

As with home health care agencies, you can expect a hospice provider to develop a written plan of care with specific duties, work hours/days, and the contact numbers of staff members you can call.

Updating the plan of care may not be crucial for most hospice patients, but check on how the plan will be amended if your loved one's needs change.

7. How do you assign people to new clients? Will you honor our preferences?

Even more important in hospice care than home health care is the need for the people around you to have pleasant, compassionate, and supportive personalities. You don't want a sourpuss blabbing on his cell phone while your loved is dying in the next room.

Good follow-up questions will help to ensure this doesn't happen to you. Ask:

- Do we have any choices in which caregiver you send?
- Can we meet the hospice caregivers in advance?
- Will you consistently send the same caregivers?
- Can we request someone else if we aren't satisfied?

ISO: A PLEASANT PERSONALITY

Special care requires special people. Experience is only a guide to a good caregiver, not a guarantee for the personality characteristics needed for hospice. Look for a person who has a sense of humor, who is cheerful, mature, caring, patient, observant, accountable, and flexible — and someone who sees you and your loved one as special people, too. You want a hospice worker who isn't condescending and treats your loved one with respect and dignity.

8. Who will supervise the quality of care for my loved one? How can I reach this person? What are your procedures for after-hours questions or concerns?

You want to be sure a responsible, professional nurse or manager is in charge and reachable at all times. Ask for the person's direct phone number, not the main switchboard number. Be sure you're clear on how to reach her after hours.

9. What are your costs, and can I have a written description of your services?

Get in writing the provider's costs, payment policies and procedures, billing timeline, and any informal offers the provider has made for financial assistance or to check on aid for you. Ask if the provider has resources to help you find financial assistance, if needed.

Medicare and private health insurance usually cover hospice care for eligible patients. Insurance or veterans' benefits may also provide financial coverage. Some hospice programs are available on a sliding fee scale based on family income.

10. Please provide me with a list of three previous clients whom I can contact for referrals.

As with the referrals for home health care agencies, ask for a list of previous clients of this hospice provider whom you can call.

See chapter 14, Best Question 10 (page 148), for a list of important questions to ask each referral.

❯ The Magic Question

How do you resolve client problems and complaints?

If you contract with a quality hospice provider, the chance of having problems, disappointments, or complaints will be small. However, you can tell how professional providers are from their readiness and willingness to tell you how they have solved past problems.

If the answer is, "We don't have problems," or the person is reluctant to discuss this topic with you, that should be a red flag. The best companies (and people) are highly aware of what they do well, how they can improve, and are candid about explaining how they learned from past problems.

To encourage more conversation, ask for an example or stories about past problems that were solved well. The best answers include being able to reach a responsible person twenty-four hours a day.

How a hospice provider responds to a test call may be a good indicator of the level of care you can expect later. Try calling the twenty-four-hour number at an off time to see how quick and compassionate their response is. Do the staffers sound professional and customer friendly, or are they sullen and focused on internal procedures and rules?

CONCLUSION

Some people feel shy or reluctant to question hospice providers closely about their services and costs. But what could be more important than ensuring that your loved one will receive top-quality care during the final phase of her life?

There are similarities between choosing a home health care agency and a hospice provider. In both cases, you want a Medicare-accredited company that provides a written, detailed plan and itemized cost list. Accreditation by a national organization is the gold standard. There are similar security, safety, and trust concerns about having strangers in your home and the need for fully screened workers. The key difference is the usual duration of the contract.

You are likely to feel emotionally fragile and conflicted as you search for hospice care. If possible, try to do your homework early. Advance planning to find a hospice provider before your loved one's condition worsens gives you more control, more choices, and helps to reduce costs.

THE 10 BEST RESOURCES

American Academy of Family Physicians. "Hospice Care." www.family doctor.org/online/famdocen/home/pat-advocacy/endoflife/250.printerview .html.

Eldercare Locator. "Hospice Care." www.eldercare.gov/eldercare/Public/ resources/fact_sheets/hospice_care.asp.

HelpGuide. "Hospice Care: Full Service Support at Home or in a Facility." www.helpguide.org/elder/hospice_care.htm.

Hospice Foundation of America. "Choosing Hospice: Questions to Ask." www.hospicefoundation.org/hospiceInfo/questions.pdf.

Hospice Net. "What Questions Should I Ask About Hospice Care?" www .hospicenet.org/html/questions.html.

Joint Commission. "Helping You Choose Quality Home Care and Hospice Services." www.jointcommission.org/GeneralPublic/Choices/hc_ome.htm.

Joint Commission. "Quality Check: Find a Health Care Organization." www.qualitycheck.org/consumer/searchQCR.aspx.

MedlinePlus. "Hospice Care." www.nlm.nih.gov/medlineplus/hospicecare .html.

National Hospice and Palliative Care Organization. "Ask Your Doctor." www.caringinfo.org/UserFiles/File/PDFs/Caregiving/asktoughques tions.pdf.

National Hospice and Palliative Care Organization. "Find a Provider." www.nhpco.org/custom/directory/main.cfm.

CONCLUSION: LIVING WELL WITH
ALZHEIMER'S DISEASE

You, interrupted. That's how the doctor's words, "It's Alzheimer's disease," affect your life and the people who you love. It's a life-changing diagnosis regardless of whether you are the person with Alzheimer's, the primary caregiver, a family member, or a friend.

Whatever your initial reaction, whatever moment or stage of your life has been interrupted by this diagnosis, and no matter who you are—you can benefit from understanding the diagnosis and eventually learning everything you can about Alzheimer's disease.

Asking Best Questions—and your own great questions—at each step of the journey is a very empowering way to overcome the harsh realities of this diagnosis. Good communication is good medicine and your most powerful ally in facing Alzheimer's disease. Being a well-informed consumer can ease your stress and pain, guide your judgment, and potentially save you money in treatment and care costs.

As America's top doctor, former Surgeon General Dr. C. Everett Koop, once told the Question Doctor, "My motto has been, 'There's no prescription I can give you more valuable than knowledge.'"

In another interview, retired Surgeon General, Rear Admiral Kenneth P. Moritsugu, echoed similar sentiments. "Patients are sometimes intimidated when they are talking with their doctors, which can have cultural or generational reasons. The generation of older people often falsely assumes that their doctors know everything and just accept what they have to say."

"Being smart" has a new definition. It's not what you know. It's what you *ask* that really matters. At each stage of this journey keep asking questions—of your doctors, yourself, and one another. The only stupid question is the one left unasked.

The Question Doctor wishes you Happy Asking and all her best.

Resources

We regret any omissions or errors on this resource list. Inclusion on this list does not imply endorsement by the publisher or the author. We defined "best resource" as the most practical and content-rich information available with an emphasis on question lists and free online access.

THE 10 VERY BEST RESOURCES

Alzheimer's Disease Education and Referral. "Welcome to the ADEAR Center." www.nia.nih.gov/Alzheimers.

Alzheimer's Association, "Publications." This page provides a portal to all fact sheets and brochures available from the Alzheimer's Association. www.alz .org/alzheimers_disease_publications.asp.

Alzheimer's Association. "Resource Lists." The association's comprehensive online library is arranged by topics and types of resources. www.alz.org/we_can_ help_resource_lists.asp.

DeBaggio, Thomas. *Losing My Mind: An Intimate Look at Life with Alzheimer's.* New York: Free Press, 2003.

Family Caregiver Alliance. "Fact Sheets and Publications." www.caregiver.org/ caregiver/jsp/publications.jsp?nodeid=345.

Healthfinder.gov. Home page. Provides links for 1,500 organizations and publications. www.healthfinder.gov.

Kuhn, Daniel. *Alzheimer's Early Stages: First Steps for Families, Friends and Caregivers.* Alameda, Calif.: Hunter House Publishers, 2003.

Mace, Nancy, and Peter Rabins. *The 36-Hour Day: A Family Guide to Caring for Persons with Alzheimer's Disease, Related Dementing Illnesses, and Memory Loss in Later Life,* 4th ed. Baltimore, Md.: The Johns Hopkins University Press, 2006.

MedlinePlus. "Alzheimer's Disease." www.nlm.nih.gov/medlineplus/alzheimers disease.html.

National Institutes of Health. "PubMed Central." Portal to a free digital archive of medical journals. www.pubmedcentral.nih.gov.

CHAPTER RESOURCES

Chapter 1 — The 10 Best Questions about a Diagnosis of Alzheimer's Disease

Administration on Aging. "Alzheimer's Disease Info: Questions to Ask the Doctor." www.aoa.gov/alz/public/alzcarefam/disease_info/questions_to_ask.asp.

Alzheimer Society of Canada. "Finding Out if It Is Alzheimer Disease." www.alzheimer.ca/english/disease/diagnosis.htm.

Alzheimer's Association. "10 Warning Signs of Alzheimer's Disease." www.alz.org/national/documents/brochure_10warnsigns.pdf.

Alzheimer's Association. "2008 Alzheimer's Disease Facts and Figures." www.alz.org/national/documents/report_alzfactsfigures2008.pdf.

Alzheimer's Association. "Early Stage Alzheimer's Disease: A Guide for Health Care Professionals." www.alz.org/documents/LB_Best_Stages.pdf.

Alzheimer's Association. "Related Dementias." www.alz.org/alzheimers_disease_related_diseases.asp.

Alzheimer's Association. "Stages of Alzheimer's." www.alz.org/AboutAD/Stages.asp.

Alzheimer's Association. "Steps to Diagnosis." www.alz.org/alzheimers_disease_steps_to_diagnosis.asp.

Alzheimer's Disease Education and Referral Center (ADEAR). "Alzheimer's Disease: Fact Sheet." www.alzheimers.nia.nih.gov.

American Academy of Neurology Foundation. "Working with Your Doctor." www.thebrainmatters.org/index.cfm?key=1.2.1.

Consumer Reports Health. "Shared Decision-Making: Working with Your Doctor." www.consumerreports.org. (Subscription required.)

Family Caregiver Alliance. "Alzheimer's Disease." www.caregiver.org/caregiver/jsp/content_node.jsp?nodeid=567.

Family Caregiver Alliance. "Alzheimer's Disease: Early Stage." www.caregiver.org/caregiver/jsp/content_node.jsp?nodeid=571.

Fisher Center for Alzheimer's Research Foundation. "Alzheimer's Diagnosis Importance." www.alzinfo.org/alzheimers-diagnosis.asp.

Gruman, Jessie. *AfterShock: What to Do When the Doctor Gives You—or Someone You Love—a Devastating Diagnosis.* New York: Walker & Company, 2007.

Mayo Clinic. "Alzheimer's Stages: How the Disease Progresses." www.mayoclinic.com/health/alzheimers-stages/AZ00041.

MerekSource. "Questions to Ask Your Doctor." www.mercksource.com/pp/us/cns/cns_patient_resources_nwhrc.jspzQzpgzEzzSzppdocszSzuszSzcnszSzcontentz SznwhrcqazSzalzheimers_diseasezPzhtml. (Select "Alzheimer's Disease" from the topic list.)

National Institute on Aging. "Alzheimer's Disease: Unraveling the Mystery." www.nia.nih.gov/NR/rdonlyres/A294D332-71A2-4866-BDD7-A0DF216D AAA4/0/Alzheimers_Disease_Unraveling_the_Mystery.pdf.

National Institute on Aging. "Understanding Stages and Symptoms of Alzheimer's Disease." www.nia.nih.gov/Alzheimers/Publications/stages.htm.

National Institute on Aging. "Working with Your Older Patient: A Clinician's Handbook." www.niapublications.org/pubs/clinicians2004/chap10.asp.

Scinto, Leonard F. M., and Kirk R. Daffner. *Early Diagnosis of Alzheimer's Disease.* Totowa, N.J.: Humana Press, 2000.

Taylor, Richard. *Alzheimer's from the Inside Out.* Baltimore, Md.: Health Professions Press, 2007.

WebMD. "Alzheimer's Disease: Making the Diagnosis." www.webmd.com/alz heimers/guide/making-diagnosis.

Chapter 2 — The 10 Best Questions to Get a Reliable Referral for a Top Alzheimer's Specialist

American Academy of Neurology Foundation. "Working with Your Doctor: Preparing for an Office Visit." www.thebrainmatters.org/index.cfm?key=1.2.3.

American Medical Association, "AMA ePhysician Profiles." www.ama-assn.org/ ama/pub/category/2672.html.

Boston Central. "Doctor Referrals." www.bostoncentral.com/healthcare/doctor_ ref.php.

Charness, Neil, and Paul J. Feltovich, Robert R. Hoffman, and K. Anders Ericsson. *The Cambridge Handbook of Expertise and Expert Performance.* Cambridge: Cambridge University Press, 2006.

Consumers' Checkbook. "Guide to Top Doctors." www.checkbook.org/doctors/ pageone.cfm. (Subscription required.)

Dowie, Jack, and Arthur Elstein. *Professional Judgment: A Reader in Clinical Decision Making.* Cambridge: Cambridge University Press, 1988.

Fadiman, Anne. *The Spirit Catches You and You Fall Down: A Hmong Child, Her American Doctors, and the Collision of Two Cultures.* New York: Farrar Straus & Giroux, 1998.

Gawande. Atul. *Better: A Surgeon's Notes on Performance.* New York: Henry Holt, 2007.

Medical Board of California. "How to Choose a Doctor." www.medbd.ca.gov/ consumer/choose_doctor.html.

MedicineNet. "How to Choose a Doctor." www.medicinenet.com/script/main/art. asp?articlekey=47649.

Montgomery, Kathryn. *How Doctors Think: Clinical Judgment and the Practice of Medicine.* New York: Oxford University Press, 2005.

Petersen, Ronald. *Mayo Clinic on Alzheimer's Disease.* Rochester, Minn.: Mayo Clinic, 2002.

Randa, Jackie. "How to Choose a Good Doctor." *Desert Dispatch* (Barstow, Calif.), June 12, 2007, www.desertdispatch.com/news/doctor_764_article.html/don_need.html.

Timmermans, Stefan, and Marc Berg. *The Gold Standard: The Challenge of Evidence-Based Medicine.* Philadelphia: Temple University Press, 2003.

Chapter 3 — The 10 Best Questions to Find a Top Alzheimer's Specialist

Alzheimer's Association. "In My Community." Searchable database of local Alzheimer's Association Offices. www.alz.org/apps/findus.asp.

American Academy of Neurology Foundation. "Working With Your Doctor: Find a Neurologist." www.thebrainmatters.org/index.cfm?key=1.2.2.

American Board of Medical Specialties. "Is Your Doctor Certified?" Board certification for doctors. www.abms.org/wc/login.aspx.

American Board of Psychiatry and Neurology. "Public." Answers consumer questions on board certification. www.abpn.com/public.htm.

American Geriatrics Society. "Health Links." www.americangeriatrics.org/links.

American Medical Association. "DoctorFinder." Lets you search a database of all licensed doctors; you must specify state in which the doctor practices. www.ama-assn.org/aps/amahg.htm.

American Psychiatric Association. "Mental Health Resources." www.psych.org/Resources/MentalHealthResources.aspx.

American Psychological Association. "Find a Psychologist." http://locator.apa.org.

Federation of State Medical Boards. "Welcome to DocInfo." www.docinfo.org.

Fisher Center for Alzheimer's Research Foundation. "Alzheimer's Disease Resources in Your Area." www.alzinfo.org/providers/doctor.aspx.

Geriatric Mental Health Foundation. "Find a Geriatric Psychiatrist." www.gmhfonline.org/gmhf/find.asp.

HealthGrades. "Research Physicians." Searchable database of doctors. www.healthgrades.com. (Charges small fee.)

National Institute on Aging. "Choosing a Doctor." www.nia.nih.gov/HealthInformation/Publications/choosing.htm.

National Institute on Aging. "NIHSeniorHealth Offers Tips on How to Talk with Your Doctor." www.nia.nih.gov/NewsAndEvents/PressReleases/PR20070726talkdoctor.htm.

National Medical Association. "Physician Locator." Database of African-American physicians. http://locator.fough3.com.

WebMD. "Alzheimer's Disease Guide." www.webmd.com/alzheimers/guide/default.htm.

Resources · 277

Whitehouse, Peter, and Daniel George. *The Myth of Alzheimer's: What You Aren't Being Told About Today's Most Dreaded Diagnosis.* New York: St. Martin's Press, 2008.

Chapter 4 — The 10 Best Questions about the Test Results for Alzheimer's Disease

About.com. "Diagnosis of Alzheimer's Disease." http://alzheimers.about.com/od/diagnosisissues/Diagnosis_of_Alzheimers_Disease.htm.

Alzheimer's Disease Research Center. "Clinical Dementia Rating." www.alzheimer.wustl.edu/cdr/default.htm.

Callone, Patricia, Connie Kudlacek, Barbara Vasiloff, Janaan Manternach, and Roger Brumback. "The Progression of Alzheimer's Disease in the Brain." In *A Caregiver's Guide to Alzheimer's Disease: 300 Tips for Making Life Easier.* New York: Demos Medical Publishing, 2005.

eMedicine. "Alzheimer's Disease." www.emedicine.com/neuro/topic13.htm. (Scroll down to "Workup.")

Grady, Denise. "Finding Alzheimer's Before a Mind Fails." *New York Times,* December 26, 2007 C1.

Harvard Health Publications. "Diagnosing Alzheimer's Disease." www.mercksource.com/ppdocs/us/cns/harvard-health-reports/MerckSHR-Alzheimers082906/sections/sect7.htm.

HealthLink. "Diagnosing Alzheimer's Disease." http://healthlink.mcw.edu/article/930974303.html.

Kurlowicz, Lenore, and Meredith Wallace. "The Mini Mental State Examination (MMSE) *Try This.* January 1999. Hartford Institute for Geriatric Nursing." www.chcr.brown.edu/MMSE.pdf.

Mayo Clinic. "CT Scan." www.mayoclinic.com/health/ct-scan/FL00065.

National Institute on Aging, "How Should I Prepare? Getting Ready for an Appointment." www.nia.nih.gov/HealthInformation/Publications/TalkingWithYourDoctor/chapter02.htm.

Smith, Patricia B., and Mary M. Kenan. *Alzheimer's for Dummies.* Hoboken, N.J.: John Wiley & Sons, 2004.

Wikipedia. "Mini-Mental State Examination." www.wikipedia.org/wiki/Mini-mental_state_examination.

Chapter 5 — The 10 Best Questions to Ask When Getting a Second Opinion

Callone, Patricia, Connie Kudlacek, Barbara Vasiloff, Janaan Manternach, and Roger Brumback. "Early to Mild Stage: Something's Gone Wrong." In *A Caregiver's Guide to Alzheimer's Disease: 300 Tips for Making Life Easier.* New York: Demos Medical Publishing, 2005.

Gladwell, Malcolm. *Blink: The Power of Thinking Without Thinking*. New York: Little, Brown, 2005.

Mace, Nancy, and Peter Rabins. "Getting Medical Help for the Person with Dementia." In *The 36-Hour Day: A Family Guide to Caring for Persons with Alzheimer Disease, Related Dementing Illnesses, and Memory Loss in Later Life*, 4th ed. Baltimore, Md.: The Johns Hopkins University Press, 2006.

University of Rochester Medical Center. "Questions to Ask If Your Doctor Recommends Tests." www.stronghealth.com/questions/Tests.html.

U.S. News and World Report, "When and How to Challenge your Doctor," May 10, 1993, p. 62.

Whitehouse, Peter, and Daniel George. "Identifying Who Needs a Prescription for Memory Loss." In *The Myth of Alzheimer's: What You Aren't Being Told About Today's Most Dreaded Diagnosis*. New York: St. Martin's Press, 2008.

wikiHow. "How to Decide What to Do." www.wikihow.com/Decide-What-to-Do.

Chapter 6 — The 10 Best Questions to Ask About Alzheimer's Drugs

Alzheimer Research Forum. "Drugs and Therapies." www.alzforum.org/dis/tre/drt/default.asp.

Alzheimer's Disease Education and Referral Center (ADEAR). "Alzheimer's Disease Medications Fact Sheet." www.nia.nih.gov/Alzheimers/Publications/medicationsfs.htm.

Alzheimer's Disease Education and Referral Center (ADEAR). "*Connections* Newsletter Index." www.alzheimers.org/pubs/conindex.htm.

American Pharmacists Association. "Pharmacy and You." www.pharmacyandyou.org.

Drugs.com. "Search Drugs Function." www.drugs.com/image_search.html.

Food and Drug Administration. "Patient Information Fact Sheets." www.fda.gov/cder/drug/infopage/antipsychotics/default.htm.

Mayo Clinic. "Treatment: Alzheimer's Disease." www.mayoclinic.com/health/alzheimers-disease/DS00161/DSECTION=7.

Mayo Clinic. "Alzheimer's Drugs Slow Progression of Disease." www.mayoclinic.com/health/alzheimers/AZ00015.

National Council on Patient Information and Education. "Make Notes and Take Notes: Helpful Steps to Avoid Medication Errors." www.talkaboutrx.org/assocdocs/TASK/269/make_notes.pdf.

National Institute on Aging, ADEAR, "What Drugs are Currently Available to Treat AD?" www.nia.nih.gov/Alzheimers/AlzheimersInformation/Treatment.

Petersen, Ronald. *Mayo Clinic on Alzheimer's Disease*. Rochester, Minn.: Mayo Clinic, 2002.

Chapter 7 — The 10 Best Questions for Brain Fitness

AARP. "Tips for a Healthy Brain." www.aarp.org/health/brain/takingcontrol/tips_for_a_healthy_brain.html.

Alternative Therapies in Health and Medicine. Online home of this medical journal (subscription required). www.alternative-therapies.com.

Alzheimer's Association. "Alternative Treatments." www.alz.org/alzheimers_disease_alternative_treatments.asp.

Alzheimer's Australia. "Dementia and Art: Tips for Art at Home." www.alzheimers.org.au/upload/ArtTips.pdf.

American Horticultural Therapy Association. "The History and Practice of Horticultural Therapy." www.ahta.org/information.

American Massage Therapy Association. "Finding a Qualified Massage Therapist." www.amtamassage.org/findamassage/find.html.

American Music Therapy Association. "Music Therapy and Alzheimer's Disease." www.musictherapy.org/factsheets/MT%20Alzheimers%202006.pdf.

Burdick, Lydia. *The Sunshine on My Face: A Read-Aloud Book for Memory-Challenged Adults.* Baltimore, Md.: Health Professions Press, 2004.

Corporation for National and Community Service. "Senior Corps." www.seniorcorps.org.

Dana Foundation. "Brain Resources for Seniors." www.dana.org/resources/seniors.

Delta Society. "Search for Pet Partner Members." www.deltasociety.org/search/deltastatesearch.asp.

Elderhostel. Travel and education programs for seniors. www.elderhostel.org.

Fogler, Janet, and Lynn Stern. *Improving Your Memory: How to Remember What You're Starting to Forget.* Baltimore, Md.: The Johns Hopkins University Press, 2005.

Mackenzie, Elizabeth R., and Birgit Rakel. *Complementary and Alternative Medicine for Older Adults: Holistic Approaches to Healthy Aging.* New York: Springer, 2006.

Mayo Clinic. "Exercise and Alzheimer's: Boosts Physical and Emotional Health." www.mayoclinic.com/health/alzheimers/HQ00637.

National Center for Complementary and Alternative Medicine. "Herbs at a Glance: Ginkgo." www.nccam.nih.gov/health/ginkgo.

National Center for Creative Aging. "National Program Directory." www.creativeaging.org/programs.htm.

National Institute on Aging. "Mental Exercise Helps Maintain Some Seniors' Thinking Skills." www.nia.nih.gov/NewsandEvents/PressReleases/PR20061219ACTIVE.htm.

Snowdon, David. *Aging with Grace: What the Nun Study Teaches Us About Leading Longer, Healthier, and More Meaningful Lives.* New York: Random House, 2001.

Spencer, John W., and Joseph J. Jacobs. *Complementary and Alternative Medicine: An Evidence-Based Approach.* St. Louis, Mo.: Mosby, 2003.

Weil, Andrew. *Natural Health, Natural Medicine: The Complete Guide to Wellness and Self-Care for Optimum Health,* rev. ed. Boston: Houghton Mifflin, 2004.

Chapter 8 — The 10 Best Questions to Avoid Alternative Treatment Scams

Better Business Bureau. "For Consumers." http://us.bbb.org/WWWRoot/Site Page.aspx?site=113&id=b81f1c7b-c315-4f43-8d92-a44a2248ec44.

Consumer Healthcare Products Association. "Dietary Supplements Are Regulated Products." www.chpa-info.org/ChpaPortal/issues/DSHEA/DietarySupplements.htm

Food and Drug Administration. "MedWatch Reporting by Consumers." www.fda.gov/medwatch/report/consumer/consumer.htm.

MedlinePlus. "MedlinePlus Guide to Healthy Web Surfing." www.nlm.nih.gov/medlineplus/healthywebsurfing.html.

Milloy, Steven J. *Junk Science Judo: Self-Defense Against Health Scares and Scams.* Washington, D.C.: Cato Institute, 2001.

National Association of Boards of Pharmacy. "Boards of Pharmacy." www.nabp.net/indexroster.asp.

National Center for Complementary and Alternative Medicine. "Herbal Supplements: Consider Safety, Too." www.nccam.nih.gov/health/supplement-safety.

National Consumer's League. "For Consumers." www.nclnet.org/fraud.

National Council Against Health Fraud. Home page. www.ncahf.org.

Office of Dietary Supplements. "Health Information." www.ods.od.nih.gov/Health_Information/Health_Information.aspx.

Quackwatch. "Questionable Products, Services, and Theories." www.quackwatch.org.

U.S. Postal Inspection Service. "Mail Fraud." www.usps.com/postalinspectors/fraud.

Chapter 9 — The 10 Best Questions Before Participating in a Clinical Trial

Alzheimer's Association. "Ethical Issues in Dementia Research (with Special Emphasis on Informed Consent)." www.alz.org/national/documents/statements_ethicalissues.pdf.

Alzheimer's Association. "Participating in Clinical Trials and Research." www.alz.org/national/documents/topicsheet_clinicalstudies.pdf.

Center for Information and Study on Clinical Research Participation. "Education Before Participation." www.ciscrp.org/information/documents/2006Brochure English.pdf.

Cichocki, Mark. "Top 10 Questions to Ask About Clinical Trials." http://aids.
about.com/od/clinicaltrials/tp/trialq.htm.

Ferris, S. H. "Clinical Trials in AD: Are Current Formats and Outcome Measures
Adequate?" *Alzheimer Disease and Associated Disorders* 16 (2002): S13–S17.

Greene, Kelly. "Playing Guinea Pig: More Clinical Trials Need Older Volunteers.
Should you Raise Your Hand?" *Wall Street Journal,* August 11, 2003, C5.

Keim, Brandon. "So You Want to Be a Gene Therapy Guinea Pig?" http://blog.
wired.com/wiredscience/2007/07/so-you-want-to-.html.

International Federation of Pharmaceutical Manufacturers & Associations. "Clinical Trials Portal." Search ongoing drug trials and trial results. http://clinical
trials.ifpma.org/no_cache/en/myportal/index.htm.

"Is a Clinical Trial Right for Your Older Relative?" *Work & Family Life,* May
2003, p. 17.

MerckSource. "What Participants Need to Know About Clinical Trials." www
.mercksource.com/pp/us/cns/cns_merckmanual_frameset.jsp?pg=http://merck
.com/mmhe/sec25/ch307666/ch307666c.html.

National Institute on Aging. "Alzheimer's Disease Centers." www.nia.nih.gov/
ResearchInformation/ExtramuralPrograms/NeuroscienceOfAging/Program
Initiatives/ADC.htm.

"Questions to Ask During Clinical Trials." *Healthcare PR and Marketing News,*
November 23, 2000.

Chapter 10 — The 10 Best Questions to Decide if Your Loved One Can Remain at Home

Alternatives for Seniors. "Evaluation Tool." www.alternativesforseniors.com/Eval
uation.aspx.

Alzheimer's Association. "Coping with Changes." www.alz.org/living_with_alz
heimers_coping_with_changes.asp. (scroll down to "Living Alone.")

Alzheimer's Association. "Disaster Preparedness." www.alz.org/living_with_alz
heimers_disaster_preparedness.asp.

Amella, Elaine J. "Assessing Nutrition in Older Adults," *Try This.* Issue 9, revised
2007. Hartford Institute for Geriatric Nursing. www.hartfordign.org/publica
tions/trythis/issue_9.pdf.

American Medical Association. *American Medical Association Guide to Home Caregiving.* New York: John Wiley & Sons, 2001.

American Seniors Housing Association. "Housing Options for Seniors." http://
consumer.seniorshousing.org/housing/index.aspx.

Beverly Foundation. "Local Sources to Tap for Transportation." www.beverly
foundation.org/resourcestore/pdf/general_information/community_transporta
tion_resources.pdf.

Family Caregiver Alliance. "Caring for Adults with Cognitive and Memory Impairments." www.caregiver.org/caregiver/jsp/content_node.jsp?nodeid=392.

Gordeau, Bretten C., and Jeffrey G. Hillier. *Alzheimer's Essentials: Practical Skills for Caregivers,* 2nd ed. Lake Worth, Fla.: Carma Publishing, 2007.

Graf, Carla. "The Lawton Instrumental Activities of Daily Living (IADL) Scale." *Try This.* Issue 23, revised 2007. Hartford Institute for Geriatric Nursing. www.hartfordign.org/publications/trythis/issue23.pdf.

Mayo Clinic. "Alzheimer's: Dealing with Daily Challenges." www.mayoclinic.com/health/alzheimers/AZ00026.

Meals on Wheels Association of America. "Looking for a Meal: Find Meals Near You." www.mowaa.org/searchMealProgram.asp?MemberNo=5E5D57&CurrentNo=5E5D56&type=1

Meyer, Maria M. *The Comfort of Home: An Illustrated Step-By-Step Guide for Caregivers,* 2d. ed. Portland, Or.: Care Trust Publications, 2002.

National Association for Continence. "Frequently Asked Questions About Incontinence." www.nafc.org/bladder-bowel-health/frequently-asked-questions.

National Association of Home Builders. "Aging-in-Place Checklists." www.nahb.org/generic.aspx?sectionID=717&genericContentID=89801.

National Institute on Aging. "There's No Place Like Home—For Growing Old." www.niapublications.org/tipsheets/home.asp.

Taira, Ellen D., and Jodi L. Carlson, eds. *Aging in Place: Designing, Adapting and Enhancing the Home Environment.* London: Haworth, 2000.

University of Texas. School of Nursing at Houston. "Katz Basic Activities of Daily Living (ADL) Scale and Lawton-Brody Instrumental Activities of Daily Living Scale (IADL)." http://son.uth.tmc.edu/coa/FDGN_1/RESOURCES/ADLandIADL.pdf.

Volunteers of America. "Local Offices." www.volunteersofamerica.org/LocalOffices/tabid/5127/Default.aspx.

Chapter 11: The 10 Best Questions to Assess Home Safety for a Loved One with Alzheimer's Disease

AgeNet. "Home Safety Checklist." www.agenet.com/Category_Pages/document_display.asp?cat_id=13&id=341.

Alzheimer Society of Canada. "Safely Home," Alzheimer wandering registry. www.safelyhome.ca/en/safelyhome/safelyhome.asp.

Alzheimer's Association. "Home Safety." www.alz.org/living_with_alzheimers_home_safety.asp.

Alzheimer's Australia. "Safety Issues." www.alzheimers.org.au/content.cfm?info pageid=4525.

American Occupational Therapy Association. "Modifying Your Home for Independence." www.aota.org/Consumers/Tips/Adults/HomeMods/35132.aspx.

Ashton, Jessica. "Fear of Falling." *Caregiver,* March/April 2006. www.caregiver.com/magazine/2006/mar-apr/fear_of_falling.htm.

AssistGuide Information Services. "Home Safety and Security Checklist." www.agis.com/Document/13/home-safety-and-security-checklist.aspx.

Brawley, Elizabeth C. *Design Innovations for Aging and Alzheimer's.* New York: John Wiley & Sons, 2005.

Cohen, Uriel, and Gerald D. Weisman. *Holding on to Home: Designing Environments for People with Dementia.* Baltimore, Md.: The Johns Hopkins University Press, 1991.

Consumers' Checkbook. "Home Security." www.checkbook.org (subscription required).

Eldercare Team. "Senior Home Safety Assessment." www.eldercareteam.com/assessment/homesafety.pdf.

Home Safety Council. "Older Adult Research." www.homesafetycouncil.org/home/home_june06_w002.aspx.

Mayo Clinic. "Alzheimer's: Understand and Control Wandering." www.mayoclinic.com/health/alzheimers/HQ00218.

MedicAlert Foundation International. "MedicAlert + Safe Return." www.medicalert.org/SafeReturn.

MetLife. "Falls and Fall Prevention." www.metlife.com/WPSAssets/8846406400 1080659160V1FFalls%20and%20Fall%20Prevention%2003-04.pdf.

National Fire Protection Association. "Emergency Evacuation Planning Guide for People with Disabilities." www.nfpa.org/assets/files//PDF/Forms/Evacuation Guide.pdf.

National Hospice and Palliative Care Organization. "Home Safety." www.caringinfo.org/CaringForSomeone/PreparingForGivingCare/HomeSafety.htm.

National Institute on Aging. "Falls and Fractures." www.nia.nih.gov/Health Information/Publications/falls.htm.

National Resource Center for Safe Aging. "Resource Database." www.safeaging.org/resources/resource_search.asp.

National Safety Council. "Falls in the Home and Community." www.nsc.org/resources/issues/fallstop.aspx.

Thriving at Home. "A Safety Checklist for Your Home." www.thrivingathome.com/content/safety.shtml.

Warner, Mark, and Ellen Warner. *The Complete Guide to Alzheimer's-Proofing Your Home.* West Lafayette, Ind.: Purdue University Press, 2000.

Chapter 12: — The 10 Best Questions to Decide,
Should Mom Move In with Me?

AARP. "Involving the Whole Family in Caregiving." www.aarp.org/families/caregiving/caring_help/a2003-10-27-caregiving-wholefamily.html.

Alzheimer's Association. "Caregiver Guides." www.alz.org/national/documents/CareGuides_RL.doc.

Area Agency on Aging of Pasco-Pinellas. "The Four Stages of Caregiving." www.agingcarefl.org/caregiver/fourStages.

AXA Equitable. "Aging Parents and Common Sense: A Practical Guide for You and Your Parents." www.caregiving.org/pubs/brochures/Aging%20Parent=Guide_5thEd.pdf.

Delehanty, Hugh, and Elinor Ginzler. *Caring for Your Parents: The Complete AARP Guide.* New York: Sterling Publishers, 2006.

Eldercare. "Living Alternatives." www.eldercare.com/modules.php?op=modload&name=CG_Resources&file=index&catid=&cg_topic=8

Family Caregiver Alliance. "Selected Caregiver Statistics." www.caregiver.org/caregiver/jsp/content_node.jsp?nodeid=439.

Gould, Jean. *Dutiful Daughters: Caring for Our Parents as They Grow Old.* Seattle, Wash. Seal Press, 1999.

National Safety Council. "Tips to Help You Care for Aging Parents." www.nsc.org/resources/issues/articles/falltips.aspx.

Piver, Susan. *How Not to Be Afraid of Your Own Life.* New York: St. Martin's Press, 2007.

Rob, Caroline. "Before Your Older Relative Moves In, Ask These Questions." *Work and Family Life,* 17 (Nov. 2003): 6.

Strength for Caring. Home page. www.strengthforcaring.com/index.html.

Taylor, Dan. *The Parent Care Conversation: Six Strategies for Dealing with the Emotional and Financial Challenges of Aging Parents.* New York: Penguin, 2004.

Chapter 13 — The 10 Best Questions to Find Quality Adult Day Care
for Alzheimer's Patients

Alzheimer's Association. "Adult Day Centers." www.alz.org/national/documents/topicsheet_adultday.pdf.

ARCH National Respite Network and Resource Center. "Adult Day Care: One Form of Respite for Older Adults." www.archrespite.org/archfs54.htm.

CareGuide@Home. "Adult Day Care Checklist." www.careguideathome.com/modules.php?op=modload&name=CG_Resources&file=article&sid=1060# CareGuide's Living Alternatives.

CarePathways. "Adult Day Care." www.carepathways.com/ADCx.cfm.

Fairfax County, Virginia. "FAQ Adult Day Health Care." www.fairfaxcounty.gov/
hd/adhc/adhcfaq.htm#faq01.

Inter-Generations. "What to Look for When Choosing an Adult Day Care." www
.intergens.com/featurearticle-19.html#Inter%20Generations.

Marcell, Jacqueline. *Elder Rage, or Take My Father . . . Please! How to Survive Caring
for Aging Parents.* Irvine, Calif.:Impressive Press, 2001.

Mayo Clinic. "Sundowning: Late-day Confusion." www.mayoclinic.com/health/
sundowning/HQ01463.

MetLife. "Community Services." www.metlife.com/FileAssets/MMI/MMISYCCom
munityServices2007.pdf.

Mitchell, Rosas. "Home from Home: A Model of Daycare for People with Dementia." *Generations.* 23 (Fall 1999): 78–81.

Moore, Keith Diaz. "Design Guidelines for Adult Day Services." www.aia.org/
SiteObjects/files/Diaz_Moore_color.pdf.

Moore, Keith Diaz, Lyn Dally Geboy, and Gerald D. Weisman. *Designing a Better
Day: Guidelines for Adult and Dementia Day Services Centers.* Baltimore, Md.:
The Johns Hopkins University Press, 2006.

National Hospice and Palliative Care Organization. "Community Resources."
www.caringinfo.org/CaringForSomeone/PreparingForGivingCare/Commu
nityResources.htm.

Spinks, Martha. "Opening an Alzheimer's Day Care Center." *Nursing Homes,* 54
(April 2005): 48–53.

Chapter 14 — The 10 Best Questions to Hire a Top Home Health Care Agency

Accreditation Commission for Health Care. "What Is Accreditation?" www.achc
.org/public_accreditation.php.

AgeNet. "How to Find In-Home Care: Identifying In-Home Caregivers." www.age
net.com.

CarePathways. "Choosing Home Care; What You Should Know." www.carepath
ways.com/cto21.cfm.

FreedomEldercare. "Why Hire a Licensed Agency." www.freedomeldercare.com/
licensed-agency.asp.

Mayo Clinic. "Home Care Services: What Services Do You Need?" www.mayo
clinic.com/print/home-care-services/HA00086/METHOD=print.

Medicare. "Glossary of Definitions." www.medicare.gov/HHCompare/Static/Re
lated/GlossaryPopUp.asp.

MedlinePlus. "Home Care Services." www.nlm.nih.gov/medlineplus/homecareser
vices.html.

MetLife. "Understanding Home Care Agency Options." www.metlife.com/File
Assets/MMI/MMISYCUnderstandingHomeCare.pdf.

National Association for Home Care and Hospice. "Accrediting Agencies." www
.nahc.org/consumer/agencies.html.

National Association for Home Care and Hospice. "How Do I Select the Right
Home Care Provider?" www.nahc.org/consumer/selection.html.

National Association for Home Care and Hospice. "NAHC Agency Locator:
Looking for a Home Care or Hospice Agency?" www.nahc.org/agencylocator/
home.html.

National Family Caregiver Support Program. "How Do I Hire a Home Care
Employee?" www.aoa.gov/prof/aoaprog/caregiver/carefam/taking_care_of_
others/wecare/hire.asp.

New Horizons Un-Limited. "Guide to Searching for and Selecting a Home Health
Aide." www.new-horizons.org/gdehha.html.

Visiting Nurse Associations of America. "Choosing a Home Health Care Agency."
www.vnaa.org/vnaa/g/?H=HTML/ChoosingAHomeHealthCareAgency.html.

Chapter 15 — The 10 Best Questions to Choose a Long-Term Care Facility for an Alzheimer's Resident

AARP. "Choosing a Nursing Home." www.aarpmagazine.org/health/embedded_
sb.html.

Administration on Aging. "Long Term Care Ombudsman Program." www.aoa.
gov/eldfam/Elder_Rights/LTC/LTC.aspx.

Alzheimer's Association. "Dementia Care Practice Recommendations for Assisted
Living Residences and Nursing Homes." www.alz.org/national/documents/
brochure_DCPRphases1n2.pdf.

American Association of Colleges of Nursing. "Nursing Shortage." www.aacn
.nche.edu/Media/FactSheets/NursingShortage.htm.

American Association of Homes and Services for the Aging. "How to Choose."
www.aahsa.org/consumer_info/how_to_choose/default.asp.

American Medical Directors Association. "Quality Measures." www.amda.com/
consumers/qualitydata.cfm.

Assisted Living Federation of America. "Looking for an Assisted Living Residence?" www.alfa.org/i4a/pages/index.cfm?pageid=3267.

CarePathways. "Alzheimer's Care via Long-Term Care Facilities." www.carepath
ways.com/ALZr.cfm.

Consumer Consortium on Assisted Living. "Consumers and Care Givers." www
.ccal.org/consumers_care.htm.

Consumers Union. *Complete Guide to Health Services for Seniors.* New York: Three
Rivers Press, 2000.

Consumers Union. "Safety Alert: The Quality of Nursing-Home Care, November
2003." www.consumerreport.org. (Subscription only.)

HealthGrades.com. "Research Nursing Homes." www.healthgrades.com.

Kansas Department on Aging. "How to Select a Special Care Unit." www.aging kansas.org/Publications/SpecialCare/HowtoSelect.pdf.

Mayo Clinic. "Long Term Health Care: Plan Ahead." www.mayoclinic.com/health/ long-term-care/HA00054.

MetLife. "Choosing an Assisted Living Facility." www.metlife.com/FileAssets/ MMI/MMISYCChoosingAssistedLivingFac.pdf.

MetLife. "Making the Nursing Home Choice." www.metlife.com/FileAssets/MMI/ MMISYCNursingHomeChoice2007.pdf.

Morris, Virginia, and Robert M. Butler. "A Good Nursing Home." In *How to Care for Aging Parents.* New York: Workman Publishing, 2004.

MyZiva. "Find a Nursing Home." www.myziva.net.

National Center for Assisted Living. "Consumer Information." www.ncal.org/ consumer/index.cfm.

NCCNHR (National Citizens' Coalition for Nursing Home Reform). "A Consumer Guide to Choosing a Nursing Home." http://nccnhr.newc.com/uploads/ NhConsumerGuide.pdf.

Nursing Home Ombudsman Agency of the Bluegrass, Inc. "A Guide to Making Placement Decisions." www.ombuddy.org/InfoSheet/placement.htm.

Chapter 16 — The 10 Best Questions to Recognize Elder Abuse

Action On Elder Abuse (UK). "Helpline." www.elderabuse.org.uk/Mainpages/ Helpline.htm.

Administration on Aging. "Elder Rights: Preventing Fraud & Abuse." www.aoa .gov/eldfam/Elder_Rights/Preventing_Fraud/Preventing_Fraud.aspx.

Alzheimer's Association. "Know Residents' Rights in a Care Facility and When to Speak Up." www.alz.org/national/documents/carefinder_topicsheet_know rights.pdf.

Haworth Press. *"Journal of Elder Abuse and Neglect"* (subscription required). www .haworthpress.com/store/product.asp?sku=J084.

National Center on Elder Abuse. "Elder Abuse Prevalence and Incidence." www .ncea.aoa.gov/NCEAroot/Main_Site/pdf/publication/FinalStatistics050331.pdf.

National Center on Elder Abuse. "Forgotten Victims of Elder Financial Crime and Abuse." www.ncea.aoa.gov/NCEAroot/Main_Site/pdf/publication/fvefca.pdf.

National Center on Elder Abuse. "Nursing Home Abuse: Risk Prevention Profile and Checklist." www.ncea.aoa.gov/NCEAroot/Main_Site/pdf/publication/ NursingHomeRisk.pdf.

National Center for Elder Abuse. "State Resource Directory on Elder Abuse Prevention." www.ncea.aoa.gov/NCEAroot/Main_Site/Find_Help/State_Re sources.aspx. Abuse hotline: 1-800-677-1116.

National Citizens' Coalition for Nursing Home Reform. "Abuse and Neglect." www.nccnhr.org/public/50_156_450.cfm.

National Domestic Violence Hotline. "Break the Silence, Make the Call." www.ndvh.org. Hotline: 800-799-SAFE (7233).

National Institute on Aging. "Crime and Older People." www.nia.nih.gov/HealthInformation/Publications/crime.htm.

National Organization for Victim Assistance. "Adult Victims of Crime and Abuse in Residential Care Facilities." www.trynova.org/victiminfo/elderly.

Nursing Home Abuse Resource Center. "Resources." www.nursinghomeabuse resourcecenter.com.

University of Delaware's Clearinghouse on Abuse and Neglect of the Elderly. "Welcome!" www.cane.udel.edu/cane.

Chapter 17 — The 10 Best Questions for a Caregiver's Emotional Health

Alzheimer's Association. "Caregiver Guides." www.alz.org/national/documents/CareGuides_RL.doc.

Alzheimer's Disease Education and Referral Center. "*Connections* Newsletter Index." www.nia.nih.gov/Alzheimers/ResearchInformation/Newsletter.

Alzheimer's Foundation of America. "Behavioral Challenges: Strategies to Head Off or Deal with Behavior Problems." www.alzfdn.org/EducationandCare/strategies_pr.html.

Avadian, Brenda. *Finding the Joy in Alzheimer's: Caregivers Share the Joyful Times.* Pearblossom, Calif.: North Star Books, 2002.

Braff, Sandy, and Mary Rose Olenik. *Staying Connected While Letting Go: Alzheimer's—The Caregiver's Paradox.* New York: M. Evans and Company, 2005.

Callone, Patricia R., Barbara Vasiloff, Connie Kudlacek, Janaan Manternach, and Roger Brumback. *Alzheimer's Disease, the Dignity Within: A Handbook for Caregivers, Family and Friends.* New York: Demos Medical Publishing, 2005.

Canfield, Jack, Mark Victor Hansen, and Heather McNamara. *Chicken Soup for the Unsinkable Soul: 101 Stories.* Deerfield Beach, Fla. HCI, 1999.

Duke Family Support Program. *Lessons Learned: Shared Experiences in Coping.* Durham, N.C.: Duke University Medical Center, 1999.

Family Caregiver Alliance. "A Physician's View of Caregiver Health." www.care giver.org/caregiver/jsp/content_node.jsp?nodeid=1564.

Gruetzner, Howard. *Alzheimer's: A Caregiver's Guide and Sourcebook,* 3rd ed. New York: John Wiley & Sons, 2001.

HelpGuide. "Alzheimer's Caregivers Support." www.helpguide.org/elder/alzhei mers_disease_dementia_support_caregiver.htm.

Jacobs, Barry J. *The Emotional Survival Guide for Caregivers: Looking After Yourself and Your Family While Helping an Aging Parent.* New York: Guilford Press, 2006.

Kübler-Ross, Elisabeth. *On Grief and Grieving: Finding the Meaning of Grief Through the Five Stages of Loss.* New York: Simon & Schuster, 2005.

Kurlowicz, Lenore, and Sherry A. Greenberg. "The Geriatric Depression Scale (GDS)." *Try This.* Issue 4, revised 2007. Hartford Institute for Geriatric Nursing. www.hartfordign.org/publications/trythis/issue04.pdf.

Lotsa Helping Hands. "How It Works." www.lotsahelpinghands.com/ltc/how.

Mayo Clinic. "Depression Common Among Caregivers." www.mayoclinic.com/health/alzheimers/AZ00063.

McCann-Beranger, Judith. *A Caregiver's Guide for Alzheimer and Related Diseases.* Lancaster, Penn.: Acorn Press, 2004.

Mental Health America. "Finding Help." www.nmha.org/go/help/finding=help

Mittelman, Mary S., Cynthia Epstein, and Alicia Pierzchala. *Counseling the Alzheimer's Caregiver: A Resource for Health Care Professionals.* Chicago: American Medical Association Press, 2002.

National Alliance for Caregiving. "Welcome!" www.caregiving.org.

National Family Caregivers Association. "Caregiving Resources." www.nfcacares.org/caregiving_resources.

National Institute on Aging. "Depression: Don't Let the Blues Hang Around." www.nia.nih.gov/HealthInformation/Publications/depression.htm.

Oliver, Rose, and Frances A. Bock. *Coping with Alzheimer's: A Caregiver's Emotional Survival Guide.* Chatsworth, Calif.: Wilshire Book Company, 1989.

Seidman, Howard. "When Men Become Caregivers." www.healthatoz.com/health atoz/Atoz/common/standard/transform.jsp?requestURI=/healthatoz/Atoz/hc/men/life/caregivers.jsp.

Warnock, Sheila. *Share the Care: How to Organize a Group to Care for Someone Who Is Seriously Ill.* New York: Fireside, 2004.

Chapter 18 — The 10 Best Questions when One Spouse Has Alzheimer's Disease

Alzheimer's Association. "Changes in Relationships." www.alz.org/living_with_alzheimers_changes_in_relationships.asp.

Alzheimer's Association. "Sexuality and Intimacy Issues in Alzheimer's Disease." www.alz.org/national/documents/SexandIntimac_RL.doc. (Resource list.)

American Association for Marriage and Family Therapy. "Search for Marriage and Family Therapist Near You." www.therapistlocator.net.

American Counseling Association. "Counselor Directory." www.counseling.org/Resources/CounselorDirectory/TP/Home/CT2.aspx.

Butler, Robert N., and Myrna I. Lewis. *The New Love and Sex After 60*. New York: the Ballantine Publishing Group, 2002.

Cole, Harriette, and John Pinderhughes. *Coming Together: Celebrations for African-American Families*. New York: Jump in the Sun Publishers, 2003.

Gray, John. *Men Are from Mars, Women Are from Venus: The Classic Guide to Understanding the Opposite Sex*. New York: Harper Paperbacks, 2004.

Kessler L. *Dancing with Rose: Finding Life in the Land of Alzheimer's*. New York: Viking, 2007.

Mayo Clinic. "Alzheimer's: Dealing with Family Conflict." www.mayoclinic.com/health/alzheimers/AZ00027.

National Institute on Aging. "Study Sheds New Light on Intimate Lives of Older Americans." www.nia.nih.gov/NewsAndEvents/PressReleases/PR20070823sexlives.htm.

Peck, Scott, and Shannon Peck. *The Love You Deserve: A Spiritual Guide to Genuine Love*. Solana Beach, Calif.: Lifepath Publishing, 2002.

Reinisch, June M., and Ruth Beasley. *The Kinsey Institute New Report On Sex: What You Must Know to Be Sexually Literate*. New York: St. Martin's Press, 1990.

Well Spouse Association. "Support Groups by State." www.wellspouse.org/index.php?option=com_contxtd&Itemid=50.

Chapter 19—The 10 Best Questions for Long-Distance Caregivers— Does Dad Need Help?

AARP. "Talking to Older Parents About Independence." www.aarp.org/health/healthyliving/articles/caregiving-aboutindependence.html.

Alzheimer's Resource Room. "Long Distance Caregiving." www.aoa.gov/alz/public/alzcarefam/caregiving_tips/long_distance_care.asp.

Beerman, Susan, and Judith Rappaport-Musson. "Long-Distance Caregiving." In *Eldercare 911: The Caregiver's Complete Handbook for Making Decisions*. Amherst, N.Y.: Prometheus Books, 2008.

Berman, Claire. *Caring for Yourself While Caring for Your Aging Parents: How to Help, How to Survive*, 3rd ed. New York: Owl Books, 2006.

Canfield, Jack, Mark Victor Hansen, LeAnn Thieman, and Rosalynn Carter. *Chicken Soup for the Caregiver's Soul: Stories to Inspire Caregivers in the Home, the Community, and the World*. Deerfield Beach, Fla.: HCI, 2004.

Caring from a Distance. "Welcome." www.cfad.org.

Children of Aging Parents. "A National Organization for Caregivers." www.caps4caregivers.org.

Cohen, Donna, and Carl Eisdorfer. *The Loss of Self: A Family Resource for the Care of Alzheimer's Disease and Related Disorders*. New York: W. W. Norton & Company, 2002.

Davis, Patty. *The Long Goodbye: Memories of My Father.* New York: Knopf, 2004.

Heath, Angela. *Long Distance Caregiving: A Survival Guide for Far Away Caregivers.* New York: Amer Source Books, 1993.

Levin, Nora Jean. *How to Care for Your Parents: A Practical Guide to Eldercare.* New York: W. W. Norton, 1997.

Mayo Clinic. "Aging Parents: 10 Things to Know for an Emergency." www.mayo clinic.com/health/senior-health/HA00029.

MetLife. "Family Caregiving." www.metlife.com/FileAssets/MMI/MMISYCFam ilyCaregiving2007.pdf.

MetLife and National Alliance for Caregiving. "Resources for Caregivers, 2007." www.caregiving.org/pubs/brochures/resourcesforcaregivers07.pdf.

Morris, Virginia, and Robert M. Butler. *How to Care for Aging Parents.* New York: Workman Publishing, 2004.

National Association of Professional Geriatric Care Managers. www.caremanager .org/?NF=1.

National Caregivers Library. "Long Distance Caregiving." www.caregiverslibrary .org/Default.aspx?tabid=168.

National Institute on Aging. "How on Earth Can My Parents Afford Everything They Need?" www.nia.nih.gov/HealthInformation/Publications/LongDistance Caregiving/chapter09.htm.

Nelson, James L., and Hile L. Nelson. *Alzheimer's: Hard Questions for Families.* New York: Doubleday Dell Publishing Group, 1997.

Net of Care. "Caregiver Resource Directory." www.netofcare.org/crd/resource_ form.asp.

Sparks, Martha Evans. *Cherish the Days: Inspiration and Insight for Long-Distance Caregivers.* Indianapolis, Ind.: Wesleyan Publishing House, 2004.

Zukerman, Rachelle. *Eldercare for Dummies.* Hoboken, N.J.: John Wiley and Sons, 2003.

Chapter 20 — The 10 Best Questions before Joining an Alzheimer's Support Group

Alzheimer's Association. "Support Groups and Dementia." Resource guide. www .alz.org/national/documents/SupportGroups_RL.doc.

Children of Aging Parents. "Caregiver Guide." www.caps4caregivers.org/guide .htm.

Kurtz, Linda. *Self-help and Support Groups: A Handbook for Practitioners.* Thousand Oaks, Calif.: Sage Publications, 1997.

Mayo Clinic. "Help, Support Crucial for Caregivers." www.mayoclinic.com/ health/alzheimers-caregivers/AZ00058.

Mittelman, Mary S., Cynthia Epstein, and Alicia Pierzchala. "Support Groups for the Caregiver." In *Counseling the Alzheimer's Caregiver: A Resource for Health Care Professionals.* Chicago: American Medical Association Press, 2002.

Murphy, Catherine. "Long Distance Caregiver: Coping With Emotions." www .caregiver.com/articles/caregiver/long_distance_caregiving.htm.

National Self-Help Clearinghouse. "What Is Self-Help and How Does It Work?" www.selfhelpweb.org/what.html#what.

Schwarz, Roger. *The Skilled Facilitator,* 2nd ed. San Francisco: Jossey-Bass, 2002.

Well Spouse Foundation. "Support Programs." www.wellspouse.org/index.php? option=com_content&task=section&id=8&Itemid=37.

Yale, Robyne. *Developing Support Groups for Individuals with Early-Stage Alzheimer's Disease: Planning, Implementation, and Evaluation.* Baltimore, Md.: Health Professions Press, 1995.

Chapter 21:— The 10 Worst Questions to Ask People with Alzheimer's Disease

Allen Klein.com. "Humor and Healing-Related Links." www.allenklein.com/links.htm.

Association for Applied and Therapeutic Humor. "AATH e-Zine." www.aath.org/ezine/ezine-2008_02.html.

Bell, Virginia, and David Troxel. *A Dignified Life: The Best Friends Approach to Alzheimer's Care, A Guide for Family Caregivers.* Deerfield Beach, Fla.: Health Communications, 2002.

Birnbach, Lisa, and Patricia Marx. *1,003 Great Things About Getting Older.* Kansas City, Mo.: Andrews McMeel Publishing, 1997.

Buckman, Elcha. *The Handbook of Humor: Clinical Applications in Psychotherapy.* Malabar, Fla.: Krieger Publishing, 1994.

Davis, Boyd H. *Alzheimer Talk, Text and Context: Enhancing Communication.* New York: Palgrave Macmillan, 2005.

Family Caregiver Alliance. "Ten Tips for Communicating with a Person with Dementia." www.caregiver.org/caregiver/jsp/content_node.jsp?nodeid=391.

Hammer, Kathryn. *And How Are We Feeling Today?* Chicago: Contemporary Books, 1993.

Helitzer, Melvin. *Comedy Writing Secrets.* Cincinnati, Ohio: F + W Publications, 1992.

Jest for the Health of It "Articles by Patty Wooten." www.jesthealth.com/frame-articles.html.

Klein, Allen. *The Healing Power of Humor.* New York: Tarcher/Putnam Books, 1989.

Metcalf, C. W., and Roma Felible. *Lighten Up: Survival Skills for People Under Pressure.* New York: Perseus Books, 1992.

Neuharth, Dan. *Secrets You Keep from Yourself: How to Stop Sabotaging Your Happiness.* New York: St. Martin's Press, 2004.

Petersen, Betsy. *Voices of Alzheimer's: Courage, Humor, Hope, and Love in the Face of Dementia.* New York: Da Capo Press, 2004.

Sherman, James R. *The Magic of Humor in Caregiving.* Golden Valley, Minn.: Pathway Books, 1995.

Strauss, Claudia J. *Talking to Alzheimer's: Simple Ways to Connect When You Visit with a Family Member or Friend.* Oakland, Calif.: New Harbinger Press, 2002.

Chapter 22 — The 10 Best Questions for Deciding When to Retire from Driving

AARP. "Driver Safety." www.aarp.org/families/driver_safety.

AARP. "Understanding Senior Transportation: Report and Analysis of a Survey of Consumers Age 50+." http://assets.aarp.org/rgcenter/il/2002_04_trans port.pdf.

American Geriatrics Society. "Safe Driving for Seniors." www.americangeriatrics .org/education/forum/driving.shtml.

American Occupational Therapy Association. "Older Drivers." www.aota.org/ Consumers/Tips/Adults/OlderDrivers.aspx.

American Safety Council. "Coaching the Mature Driver." Online course. www .arrivealivedrivingschool.com/courses/view-one?course_id=496.

Centers for Disease Control and Prevention. "Older Adult Drivers: Fact Sheet." www.cdc.gov/ncipc/factsheets/older.htm.

Clark, Rod. "Making the 'Key' Decision." www.agenet.com.

Community Transportation Association. "*CT* Magazine." http://web1.ctaa.org/ webmodules/webarticles/anmviewer.asp?a=26&z=2.

Family Caregiver Alliance. "Dementia and Driving." www.caregiver.org/caregiver/ jsp/content_node.jsp?nodeid=432.

Federal Transit Administration. "Regional Offices." www.fta.dot.gov/regional_ offices.html.

Full Circle of Care. "Driving Safety as a Family Member Ages." www.fullcirclecare .org/caregiverissues/general/driving.html.

The Hartford. " 'Getting There' Worksheet." www.thehartford.com/talkwitholder drivers/worksheets/gettingthere2.pdf.

Insurance Institute for Highway Safety. "Fatality Facts 2006: Older People." www .iihs.org/research/fatality_facts_2006_olderpeople.html.

ITNAmerica. "Overview." www.itnamerica.org/content/Overview.aspx.

Mayo Clinic. "Alzheimer's: When to Stop Driving." www.mayoclinic.com/health/ alzheimers/HO00046.

National Association of Area Agencies on Aging. "Older Driver Safety Project." www.n4a.org/older_driver_safety.

National Highway Traffic Safety Administration. "Driving and Alzheimer's Disease." www.nhtsa.dot.gov/people/injury/olddrive/Alzheimers.

National Institute on Aging. "Older Drivers." www.nia.nih.gov/HealthInformation/Publications/drivers.htm.

Roadway Safety Foundation. "Roadway Safety Guide." www.roadwaysafety.org/toc.html.

Russo, Francine. "Driving Us Crazy." *Time*, August 8, 2005, www.time.com/printout/0,8816,1090887,00.html.

SeniorDrivers.org. "Giving Up the Keys: For Families and Individuals." www.seniordrivers.org/notdriving/notdriving.cfm.

Taxicab, Limousine and Paratransit Association. "Find a Ride." www.tlpa.org/findaride/index.cfm.

USA.gov. "Senior Citizens' Resources." www.usa.gov/Topics/Seniors.shtml.

Chapter 23 — The 10 Best Questions for a Caregiver's Financial Health

Aging with Dignity. "Five Wishes." www.agingwithdignity.org/5wishes.html.

Alzheimer's Association. "Planning Ahead for Long-Term Care Expenses." www.alz.org/national/documents/topicsheet_planahead.pdf.

American Bar Association. "Commission on Law and Aging." www.abanet.org/aging.

American Geriatrics Society. "Advance Care Planning and Advance Directives." www.healthinaging.org/public_education/pef/advance_directives.php.

Burns, Sharon, and Raymond Forgue. *How to Care for Your Parents' Money While Caring for Your Parents*. New York: McGraw-Hill, 2003.

CNNMoney.com. "Personal Finance: Debt Reduction Planner." http://cgi.money.cnn.com/tools/debtplanner/debtplanner.jsp.

Employee Benefits Security Administration. www.dol.gov/ebsa.

FinanceAdvocate.com. "Links for Seniors." www.financeadvocate.com/senior.htm.

Healthwell Foundation. "Helping Patients Afford the Medical Treatments They Need." www.healthwellfoundation.org/index.aspx.

National Foundation for Credit Counseling. Consumer debt advice. www.debtadvice.org.

National Hospice and Palliative Care Organization. "Planning Ahead: Financial Information." www.caringinfo.org/PlanningAhead/FinancialInformation.htm.

National Institute on Aging. "Getting Your Affairs in Order." www.nia.nih.gov/HealthInformation/Publications/affairs.htm.

Partnership for Prescription Assistance. Searchable databases for patient and care giver programs. www.pparx.org.

Patient Access Network Foundation. "How to Apply." www.patientaccessnetwork .org/HowApply.aspx.

Patient Advocate Foundation. www.patientadvocate.org.

Pension Rights Center. "Promoting Retirement Security." www.pensionrights.org.

Social Security Administration. "Social Security Online." www.ssa.gov.

Chapter 24 — The 10 Best Questions to Settle Legal Issues at the End of Life

AARP. "Estate Planning Guide." www.aarp.org/families/end_life/a2003-12-04-endoflife-guide.html.

AARP. "Financial Powers of Attorney." www.aarp.org/families/end_life/a2003-12-02-endoflife-financialpower.html.

AARP. "Resources on End of Life, Living Wills, Dying and Death." www.aarp.org/families/end_life/recent_resources_on_end_of_life_living_wills_dying.html.

Administration on Aging. "Legal Assistance." www.aoa.gov/eldfam/Elder_Rights/Legal_Assistance/Legal_Assistance.aspx.

Alzheimer's Association. "Legal Issues." www.alz.org/living_with_alzheimers_legal_issues.asp.

Alzheimer's Australia. "Legal Planning and Dementia." www.alzheimers.org.au/upload/LegalPlanning.pdf.

American Bar Association. "Commission on Law and Aging." www.abanet.org/aging.

American Bar Association. "Consumers' Guide to Legal Help." www.abanet.org/legalservices/findlegalhelp/home.cfm.

American Bar Association. "Senior Lawyers Division." www.abanet.org/srlawyers.

American Hospice Foundation. "Legal Issues." www.americanhospice.org/index.php?option=com_content&task=blogcategory&id=19&Itemid=42.

Center for Social Gerontology. "Law and Aging." www.tcsg.org.

Center for Social Gerontology. "Links to Legal Services Providers for Older Americans." www.tcsg.org/lslinks.htm.

Consumers Union. "Final Arrangements." *Consumer Reports*, May 2001, 39.

Dippel, Raye Lynne, and J. Thomas Hutton. *Caring for the Alzheimer Patient: A Practical Guide.* Amherst, N.Y.: Prometheus Books, 1996.

ExpertLaw. "Legal Help, Information, and Resources." www.expertlaw.com.

Family Caregiver Alliance. "Durable Powers of Attorney and Revocable Living Trusts." www.caregiver.org/caregiver/jsp/content_node.jsp?nodeid=434.

Family Caregiver Alliance. "End-of-Life Decision-Making." www.caregiver.org/caregiver/jsp/content_node.jsp?nodeid=401.

Family Caregiver Alliance. "Legal Issues in Planning for Incapacity." www.care giver.org/caregiver/jsp/content_node.jsp?nodeid=437.

FindLaw. "Find a Lawyer." www.findlaw.com.

Hanks, Liza Weiman. *The Busy Family's Guide to Estate Planning: 10 Steps to Peace of Mind.* Berkeley, Calif.: Nolo Press, 2007.

H.E.L.P. "Legal Information." www.help4srs.org/legal/legalintro.htm.

Loverde, Joy. *The Complete Eldercare Planner: Where to Start, Which Questions to Ask, and How to Find Help.* 2nd ed. New York: Three Rivers Press, 2000.

Mayo Clinic. "Anticipating End-of-life Needs of People with Alzheimer's Disease." www.mayoclinic.com/health/alzheimers/HQ00618.

MedlinePlus. "Advance Directives." www.nlm.nih.gov/medlineplus/advancedirec tives.html.

National Academy of Elder Law Attorneys. "Locate an Elder Law Attorney." http:// naela.ebiz.uapps.net/solutionsite/Default.aspx?tabid=148.

National Association of State Units on Aging. "State Action on Elder Rights." www.nasua.org/elderrights.php.

National Bar Association. "The NBA Perspective." www.nationalbar.org/about/ index.shtml.

National Consumer Law Center. "Older Consumers." www.consumerlaw.org/ issues/seniors_initiative/index.shtml.

National Elder Law Foundation. "Your Lawyer and Accredited Specialist Certifi- cation." www.nelf.org/yourlawy.htm.

National Guardianship Association. "Guardianship Resources." www.guardianship .org/guardianshipResources.htm.

National Hospice and Palliative Care Organization. "Artificial Nutrition (Food) . and Hydration (Fluids) at the End of Life." www.caringinfo.org/UserFiles/ File/PDFs/ArtificialNutritionAndHydration.pdf.

National Hospice and Palliative Care Organization. "Planning Ahead." www .caringinfo.org/PlanningAhead.

National Institute on Aging. "Dementia at the End of Life." www.nia.nih.gov/ HealthInformation/Publications/endoflife/03_dementia.htm.htm.

National Senior Citizens Law Center. "Publications." www.nsclc.org/publications.

Nolo. "Conservatorships and Guardianships." www.nolo.com.siteIncludes/printer friendly.cfm/objectID/B8AFEE68-961F-4EE5-AA3E6EFD9BAEF25B/catID/ F54137F4-0641-4369-BDFD94E003B33C55/ 118/207/301/ART.

Nolo. "Elder Care: Helping a Loved One Make a Power of Attorney." www.nolo .com/resource.cfm/catID/F54137F4-0641-4369-BDFD94E003B33C55/118 /207/301.

Nolo. "Medical Powers of Attorney and Living Wills." www.nolo.com/resource .cfm/catID/EDC82D5A-7723-4A77=9E10DDB947D1F801/309/292/295.

Sargent Shriver National Center on Poverty Law. "Poverty Law Library." www
.povertylaw.org/poverty-law-library.

"Advance Directives." www.emedicinehealth.com/script/main/art.asp?articlekey
=58715&pf=3&page=1.

Chapter 25—The 10 Best Questions for Choosing Quality Hospice Care

AARP. "Hospice for End of Life Care." www.aarp.org/families/end_life/a2003-12-
02-endoflife-hospice.html.

Administration on Aging. "Hospice and Palliative Care." www.aoa.gov/prof/
notes/Docs/Hospice%20and%20Palliative%20Care.doc.

Alzheimer's Association. "Medicare's Hospice Benefit: Frequently Asked Questions." www.alz.org/national/documents/medicare_topicsheet_hospice-bene
fit.pdf.

American Association of Homes and Services for the Aging. "End-of-Life Care
Options." www2.aahsa.org/consumer_info/how_to_choose/end_of_life.asp.

American Association of Homes and Services for the Aging. "Homes and Services
Directory." www.aahsa.org/consumer_info/homes_svcs_directory/default.asp.

American Geriatric Society. "Patient Education Forum: Advance Care Planning
and Advance Directives." www.healthinaging.org/public_education/pef/
advance _directives.php.

American Hospice Foundation. "Articles." www.americanhospice.org/index.php?
option=com_content&task=blogsection&id=3&Itemid=8.

American Hospice Foundation. "Publications and Products." www.americanhos
pice.org/index.php?option=com_wrapper&Itemid=16.

Boltz, Marie. "Assessing Family Preferences for Participation in Care in Hospital-
ized Older Adults." *Try This.* Issue 22, 2007. Hartford Institute for Geriatric
Nursing. www.hartfordign.org/publications/trythis/issue22.pdf.

Doka, Kenneth. *Caregiving and Loss: Family Needs, Professional Responses.* Washington, D.C.: Hospice Foundation of America, 2001.

Doka, Kenneth. *Living with Grief: Alzheimer's Disease.* Washington, D.C.: Hospice
Foundation of America, 2004.

DyingWell.org. www.dyingwell.org.

ElderCare Online. "Hospice Benefits from Medicare." www.ec-online.net/Know
ledge/Articles/medicarehospice.html.

Glavan, Denise, Cindy Longanacre, and John Spivey. *Hospice, a Labor of Love.*
St. Louis, Mo.: Chalice Press, 1999.

GriefNet. Home page. www.griefnet.org.

Growth House. "Hospice and Home Care." www.growthhouse.org/hospice.html.

Hospice Association of America. "Consumer Information." www.nahc.org/HAA/
consumer.html.

Hospice Foundation of America. "Choosing Hospice: A Consumers Guide." Brochure ordering information. http://store.hospicefoundation.org/product.php?productid=9&cat=3&page=1.

Hospice Foundation of America. "End of Life Info." www.hospicefoundation.org/endOfLifeInfo.

Hospice Foundation of America. "Choosing Hospice: Questions to Ask." www.hospicefoundation.org/hospiceInfo/questions.pdf.

Hospice Foundation of America. "Meuser and Marwit Caregiver Grief Inventory." www.hospicefoundation.org/teleconference/2004/documents/assessment.pdf.

Hospice Foundation of America. "Welcome to the Caregiver's Corner." www.hospicefoundation.org/caregivers.

Hospice Foundation of America. "What is Hospice?" www.hospicefoundation.org/hospiceInfo.

Hospice Net. "What Questions Should I Ask About Hospice Care?" www.hospicenet.org/html/questions.html.

JAMA. "Palliative Care." http://jama.ama-assn.org/cgi/content/full/296/11/1428.

Kessler, David. *The Needs of the Dying: A Guide for Bringing Hope, Comfort, and Love to Life's Final Chapter.* New York: HarperCollins, 2007.

Knowlton, Leslie. "Hospice and Alzheimer's Disease." *Geriatric Times* (November-December 2000), www.geriatrictimes.com/g001229.html.

Mayo Clinic. "End of Life: Caring for Your Dying Loved One." www.mayoclinic.com/health/cancer/CA00048.

Mayo Clinic. "Hospice Care: An Option when Confronting Terminal Illness." www.mayoclinic.com/health/hospice-care/HQ00860.

MetLife. "Hospice Care." www.metlife.com/FileAssets/MMI/MMISYCHospice.pdf.

National Association for Home Care and Hospice. "Accrediting Agencies." www.nahc.org/consumer/agencies.html.

National Association for Home Care and Hospice. "Consumer Information." www.nahc.org/consumer/home.html.

National Association for Home Care and Hospice. "How Do I Select the Right Home Care Provider?" www.nahc.org/consumer/selection.html.

National Association for Home Care and Hospice. "NAHC Agency Locator: Looking for a Home Care or Hospice Agency?" www.nahc.org/agencylocator/home.html.

National Association for Home Care and Hospice. "What Are My Rights as a Patient?" www.nahc.org/consumer/rights.html.

National Association for Home Care and Hospice. "What Are the Standard Billing and Payment Practices?" www.nahc.org/consumer/billing.html.

National Hospice and Palliative Care Organization. "Offering Spiritual Support for Family or Friends" www.caringinfo.org/UserFiles/File/faith_brochure.pdf.

Paralyzed Veterans of America. "Veterans Benefits Department." www.pva.org/site/PageServer?pagename=benefits_main.

Post, Stephen Garrard. *The Moral Challenge of Alzheimer Disease: Ethical Issues from Diagnosis to Dying.* Baltimore, Md.: The Johns Hopkins University Press, 2002.

Sankar, Andrea. *Dying at Home: A Family Guide for Caregiving.* Baltimore, Md.: The Johns Hopkins University Press, 1999.

Silverstone, Barbara, and Helen Kandel Hyman. *You and Your Aging Parent: A Family Guide to Emotional, Social, Health, and Financial Problems.* New York: Oxford University Press, 2008.

Meet the Experts

The author interviewed each of the following experts for this book.

Clare Absher, R.N., B.S.N., of Kitty Hawk, North Carolina has thirty years' experience caring for elderly patients in assisted living and retirement homes, as a home health nurse and as a manager of a community-based home care agency. Her geriatric nursing expertise includes developing plans of care, performing needs assessments, and counseling families on care choices for their loved ones. Her Web site is www.carepathways.com.

Stephen Barrett, M.D., a retired psychiatrist in Allentown, Pennsylvania, is an author, editor, and consumer advocate best known for his popular Web site, Quackwatch. Quackwatch Inc. is a nonprofit organization whose mission is to "combat health-related frauds, myths, fads, fallacies, and misconduct" while providing "quackery-related information that is difficult or impossible to get elsewhere." His Web site is www.quackwatch.org.

Hamilton Beazley, Ph.D., is the scholar-in-residence at St. Edward's University in Austin, Texas, and author of *No Regrets: A Ten-Step Program for Living in the Present and Leaving the Past Behind*. Dr. Beazley has been interviewed on *Oprah*, NBC, CNN, and many other television and radio shows and networks. The Web site is www.stedwards.edu.

Norman Berk is a Certified Financial Planner, CPA, personal financial specialist, and J.D. and the founder of Professional Asset Strategies, LLC., in Birmingham, Alabama. Both he and his wife are cancer survivors. Mr. Berk founded a charitable organization called the Breast Cancer Research Foundation of Alabama and is on the professional advisory board of breastcancer.org. His Web site is http://proassetsllc.com.

Lorraine Biros, LCPC, is a licensed clinical professional counselor and the director for client services at the Mautner Project, The National Lesbian Health Organization, in Washington, D.C. The Mautner Project provides support for lesbians with chronic health conditions, their partners, and caregivers. Ms. Biros has more than twenty-eight years counseling experience in the lesbian and gay community. The organization's Web site is www.mautner project.org.

Peter Block has an international reputation as a management consultant and is the author of bestselling books, including *Flawless Consulting: A Guide to Getting Your Expertise Used* and *The Answer to How Is Yes*, a book that examines the underlying assumptions about asking questions. His newest book is *Community: The Structure of Belonging*, and his Web site is www.peterblock.com.

Roger A. Brumback, M. D., is the chairman of the pathology department and a professor of pathology and psychiatry at the Creighton University School of Medicine in Omaha, Nebraska. His twenty-five years of experience includes the extensive research and treatment of neurological diseases including dementia and active involvement with Alzheimer's groups. Dr. Brumback is a co-author of *Alzheimer's Disease, The Dignity Within: A Handbook for Caregivers, Family, and Friends* (2005) as well as many other popular books and academic journal articles. The Web site is www.creighton.edu.

Patricia R. Callone, M.A., M.R.E., has extensive hands-on knowledge about Alzheimer's after spending eighteen years as a caregiver to three people in her family. She co-authored *Alzheimer's Disease, The Dignity Within: A Handbook for Caregivers, Family, and Friends* (2005) and *A Caregiver's Guide to Alzheimer's Disease: 300 Tips for Making Life Easier* (2005). Ms. Callone works at Creighton University as the director of institutional and community relations for the Study of Violence Across the Lifespan. She is co-owner of CaringConcepts, Inc., founded in 2001. The Web site is www.caringconcepts.org.

Harriette Cole is a professional life coach, has authored several books, and reaches a broad multiethnic audience with her nationally syndicated advice column *Sense and Sensitivity*. Ms. Cole is currently the creative director of *Ebony* magazine. She is also the president and creative director of Harriette Cole Productions and coaches recording artists, including notable musicians such as JoJo, Alicia Keys, and Mary J. Blige. Her Web site is www.harriettecole.com. and her Wikipedia entry is at http://en.wikipedia.org/wiki/Harriette_Cole.

Linda Dano is one of daytime television's most beloved stars, best known for her Emmy-winning role as Felicia Gallant on *Another World* while simultaneously hosting Lifetime Television's *Attitudes*. She made television history playing the same character, Dr. Rae Cummings, on ABC shows *One Life to Live, All My Children, General Hospital,* and *Port Charles*. Other credits include *As the World Turns, Guiding Light,* and many other television and movie roles. In addition, she is bestselling author and businesswoman. After her father battled Alzheimer's disease, Ms. Dano became an active supporter of caregiver programs. Her Web site is www.lindadano.com and her Wikipedia entry is http://en.wikipedia.org/wiki/Linda_Dano.

Mark Gorkin, MSW, LICSW, is a licensed clinical social worker who calls himself "The Stress Doc." Mr. Gorkin is an acclaimed motivational speaker, humorist, organizational consultant, and the author of two books, *Practice Safe Stress: Healing and Laughing in the Face of Stress, Burnout and Depression* and *The Four Faces of Anger: Transforming Anger, Rage and Conflict into Inspiring Attitude and Behavior.* His Web site is www.stressdoc.com.

Neill R. Graff-Radford, M.D. is a professor of neurology at the world-famous Mayo Clinic in Jacksonville, Florida. His research interests are in degenerative neurology and dementia. He has been involved in this field since 1981, including eighteen years at the Mayo Clinic. Dr. Graff-Radford is currently the director of the Mayo group studying Alzheimer's disease. The Web site is www.mayoclinic.org.

John Gray, Ph.D., is the world's number-one-selling relationship author. An international gender and relationship expert, his *NY Times* bestselling *Men Are from Mars, Women Are from Venus* has sold more than 30 million copies worldwide. His internationally acclaimed Mars-Venus principles have helped millions of couples understand the differences between men and women. Dr. Gray's latest book, *Why Mars and Venus Collide,* is available at www.marsvenus.com/collide.

Julia R. Heiman, Ph.D., is the director of the famous Kinsey Institute for Research in Sex, Gender and Reproduction at Indiana University in Bloomington, Indiana. For more than sixty years the Kinsey Institute has been the worldwide pioneer and leader in studying human sexuality, gender, and reproduction research. Dr. Heiman's research interests include sexual arousal and traumatic sexual experiences. The Web site is www.kinseyinstitute.org.

Dale Johnson, B.S. is the executive director for the long-term care accreditation program at The Joint Commission, the premier organization responsible for assessing and accrediting U.S. hospitals and long-term care facilities. Mr. Johnson oversees all accreditation activities related to long-term care services, including the development of standards. Previously, Mr. Johnson held financial management positions in several long-term care, skilled nursing, and acute care facilities. The commission's Web site is www.jointcommission.org.

Richard Koonce is president of Richard Koonce Productions, Inc., a human resources consulting and communications firm in Brookline, Massachusetts. Mr. Koonce is an experienced writer, consultant, facilitator, coach, and interviewer and has authored four business books. His Web site is www.richardkoonce.com.

C. Everett Koop, M.D., was the U.S. Surgeon General from 1982 to 1989. He is recipient of numerous awards, including seventeen honorary doctorate degrees and the Presidential Medal of Freedom. Still going strong at 90-plus years old, Dr. Koop stays current with medical education and patient care issues. During his tenure as a high-profile Surgeon General and throughout his long career, Dr. Koop has been an outspoken advocate for improving patient-physician communications. His Wikipedia biography is at http://en.wikipe dia.org/wiki/C._Everett_Koop.

Daniel Kuhn, M.S.W., is the author of the book *Alzheimer's Early Stages: First Steps for Family, Friends and Caregivers,* 2nd edition, as well as the director of the Professional Training Institute at the Greater Illinois Chapter of the Alzheimer's Association in Chicago. Mr. Kuhn has more than thirty years experience in health care and aging, including serving as a past member of the board of directors for the American Society on Aging. The Web site is www.alz.org/illinois.

Jacqueline Marcell is the author of the bestselling book *Elder Rage, or Take My Father . . . Please!* Ms. Marcell's heart-wrenching experience as a caregiver for her elderly parents (both with Alzheimer's) propelled her to become a national speaker, radio show host, and eldercare advocate featured on CNN and in *AARP* and *Woman's Day* magazines. Her book received more than fifty endorsements from notables such as Hugh Downs and Regis Philbin. Ms. Marcell was honored as the Advocate of the Year by the National Association of Business Owners. Her Web site is www.elderrage.com.

Elaine Marshall, M.S., of Leesburg, Virginia, brought her mother into her home three years ago to care for her, despite her mother's worsening Alzheimer's symptoms and the fact that Ms. Marshall has four teenage sons. Her personal experience with Alzheimer's disease has inspired her to seek new outlets for sharing her lessons and reflections. Ms. Marshall has a master's degree in computer science and a background working with educational institutions.

Cicily Carson Maton is a Certified Financial Planner and the founder of Aequus Wealth Management Resources, a Chicago-based financial planning and investment firm that specializes in advising people during major life transitions. She has appeared several times on the television show, "Right on the Money." Her Web site is www.aequuswealth.com.

Rear Admiral Kenneth P. Moritsugu, M.D., M.P.H., retired in 2007 as the acting U.S. Surgeon General. Admiral Moritsugu's forty-year career in public health service includes many honors, including service as an Assistant Surgeon General beginning in 1988 and as Deputy Surgeon General for nearly ten years. Admiral Moritsugu's Wikipedia biography is at http://en.wikipe dia.org/wiki/Kenneth_P_Moritsugu. The U.S. Surgeon General's Web site is www.surgeongeneral.gov.

Laura Nichols, M.S., director of the Northern Virginia Long-Term Care Ombudsman Program, has nearly ten year's experience in this field, in addition to a background working for the Fairfax County Area Agency on Aging and other county government service. Ms. Nichols served for thirteen years in the

Army Reserve as an Army Medical Corp officer and earned her master's degree in counseling psychology. The Web site is www.fairfaxcounty.gov/LTCOm budsman.

Debbie Nigro is an award-winning radio personality, champion of women, author, speaker, and business executive based in New York. Ms. Nigro has interviewed hundreds of people for her radio shows, which are aired in 450 markets. She is also a consultant to the producers of the Broadway show *The First Wives Club Musical*. Ms. Nigro's video, posts, and blogs are available at www.first wivesworld.com.

Dr. Scott Peck and Shannon Peck of San Diego, California, are the cofounders of TheLoveCenter, an educational organization whose mission is to raise relationship and spiritual awareness; cohosts of a national radio show, *Love Talk*; and co-authors of several love and relationship books, including *The Love You Deserve: A Spiritual Guide to Genuine Love*. Their Web site is www.thelove center.com.

Vicki Rackner, M.D. is a board-certified surgeon who left the operating room to help patients, patients' families, and caregivers to partner more effectively with their doctors through her company, Medical Bridges. She is also an author, speaker, and consultant, including co-authoring a *Chicken Soup for the Soul: Healthy Living Series* book and several patient self-help books. Her Web site is www.medicalbridges.com.

Susan Sikora hosts a locally produced TV talk show in the San Francisco, California, area called *Bay Area Focus with Susan Sikora* and has interviewed hundreds of political, entertainment, and health celebrities on her show. Ms. Sikora is an Emmy winner who has formerly hosted live TV talk shows for PBS, CBS, NBC, and ABC. The Web site is http://cwbayarea.com.

Gary Small, M.D., is the director of UCLA's Memory and Aging Center and the author of the popular books *The Memory Bible* and *The Longevity Bible*. He is considered one of the world's foremost authorities on memory and aging. Dr. Small advocates enhancing memory performance with his self-tests and puzzles and recommends brain-saving lifestyle changes in his many publications and presentations to groups, ranging from AARP to academic conferences. His Web site is www.DrGarySmall.com.

Richard Stoltz, Ph.D., CAPT, USN, has been a mental health professional for over thirty years. During his twenty-two-year career in the Navy he has served in numerous administrative and clinical capacities. He currently serves as the assistant chief of staff at the U.S. Navy's Bureau of Medicine and Surgery.

Claudia J. Strauss writes and consults on workplace and relationship issues related to illnesses. Her book *Talking to Alzheimer's: Simple Ways to Connect When You Visit with a Family Member or Friend* launched a series on how to sustain relationships for specific health challenges. Ms. Strauss teaches business communications and public speaking at Albright College in Reading, Pennsylvania.

Helen Thomas is a legendary question asker, news service reporter, Hearst Newspapers columnist, and member of the White House press corps. She served for fifty-seven years as a correspondent and White House bureau chief for United Press International. Ms. Thomas has covered every president since John F. Kennedy and is famous for challenging presidents from her front row seat during press conferences. Ms. Thomas's Wikipedia biography is at http://en.wikipedia.org/wiki/Helen_Thomas.

Peter J. Whitehouse, M.D., Ph.D. is the co-author of the 2008 book *The Myth of Alzheimer's: What You Aren't Being Told About Today's Most Dreaded Diagnosis* (www.themythofalzheimers.com). Dr. Whitehouse is also a professor at Case Western Reserve University's Memory and Cognition Center where he specializes in neurology, geriatrics, cognitive neuroscience, and ethics. He has organized worldwide research projects on Alzheimer's drugs and edited several international Alzheimer's journals. Dr. Whitehouse co-founded The Intergenerational School (www.tisonline.org), where people with impaired memories help urban children.

Jim Winter (CDR USN, Ret.) is the director of Safety Leaders Group, a Perth, Western Australia, based company with offices in Austin, Texas, and Calgary, Alberta. Safety Leaders Group works with engineering companies to develop their leadership practices and workforce safety. Mr. Winter cares for his mother (diagnosed in 2002) who lives in Atlanta, Georgia, 11,349 miles away from his home. His Web site is www.safetyleadersgroup.com.

Paul Yurachek is a Certified Financial Planner, attorney, CPA, and a senior financial advisor with Gurtz, Yuracheck and Associates, a financial advisory practice of Ameriprise Financial Services in Bethesda, Maryland. Mr. Yurachek is a former employee of the Internal Revenue Service and has headed his own financial planning firm since 1982, specializing in retirement planning, tax planning, and estate planning.

Index

Nightingale, Florence, 142
Nigro, Debbie, 2–3
No Regrets: A Ten-Step Program for Living in the Present and Leaving the Past Behind (Beazley), 125, 257
Normal pressure hydrocephalus, 12
Northern Virginia Long-Term Care Ombudsman Program, 153
Numbers, 8
Nurses, 100, 142, 261, 264
Nursing homes, 127, 220
  cost of, 100, 161–62, 242
  dedicated Alzheimer's unit, 156
  see also Long-term care
Nutrition. *See* Diet and Nutrition
Nuts, 69

Occupational therapists, 100, 142
Oh, the Places You'll Go (Seuss), 112
Ohio State University, 29
Omega-3 fatty acids, 69, 70
On Death and Dying (Kübler-Ross), 183, 184, 186
Online groups, 211, 212, 215
Organ donation, 250
Organic foods, 72
Outbursts, 59

Painting, 105
Parkinson's disease, 11
Parents with Alzheimer's disease, 123–30, 198–207
  visits with, 159, 205
Partners with Alzheimer's disease, 189–97
Patient Bill of Rights, 145
Peck, Scott, 191
Peck, Shannon, 191
Pensions, 240
Personality, 9, 13
Personal hygiene, 102, 205
Personal laundry, 104–05
Personal property, 241
Pets, pet therapies, 54, 68, 159
PET scans (positron emission tomography), 42
Phase I trials, 87

Phase II trials, 87
Phase III trials, 87
Phase IV trials, 87–88
Physical examination, 38, 40–41
Physical history, 46
Physical outbursts, 40
Physical restraints, 172
Physical therapists, 142
Physicians. *See* Doctors
Phytochemicals, 69
Picasso, Pablo, 131
Pick's disease, 11
Place, forgetting of, 8, 12, 41
  See also Wandering
Placebos, 86
Planning for the Future, 225–69
Plastics, 72
Poison, 117, 119–20
Power of attorney, 254–55
  medical, 252
Preclinical studies, 87
Pressure sores, 170
Professional Asset Strategies, 243
Proxy, 254
Psychiatrists, 16
Psychologists, 16, 20
PubMed Central, 34
Pulse, 40, 142
Puzzles, 54

Quackwatch, 78
Question Doctor, 11, 17, 24, 30, 32, 39, 52, 55, 60, 72, 78, 94, 101, 121, 124, 135, 147, 169, 183, 190, 200, 213, 221, 236, 252, 263
Questions:
  how to ask, 1–4, 11, 17, 24, 30, 39, 60, 78, 101, 124, 147, 169, 190, 200, 221, 236, 252
  importance of, xi–xv, 1–4, 5, 8
  open vs. closed, 8, 221

Rabins, Peter, 131
Rackner, Vicki, 48–49
Razadyne, 60
Reaction times, 230
Reading, 230